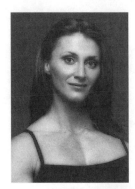

Fat or Fiction

Once upon a time, a beautiful young lady was visiting a romantic country far, far from her home. While she was there she met a wonderful young man who whisked her away to an even more romantic country, where they married and now live for six months a year. Sounds like a fairytale, but it is true!

In 1997, Donna was flown to Switzerland to train a client, and there she met her future husband, whom she married in the Bahamas the following year. They now live most of the year in Melbourne and the rest in the Bahamas.

More than ten years ago, Donna began her search for the most effective, healthy and successful way for the average person to achieve the body he or she has dreamed of. She devoured every publication and research document that she could get her hands on and she gleaned and sifted and refined, and experimented with her knowledge in her capacity as a much sought-after fitness trainer and weight-control consultant.

Along the way she put what she had learned into practice, winning a number of fitness and bodyshaping titles in Australia, which culminated in an Australian National Competition and earned her the honor of being the first Australian to gain professional status.

She has competed in a number of world bodyshaping competitions with fabulous results and will be representing Australia at the Ms Universe Competition (in the bodyshaping section) in England just as this book is 'hot off the press'!

Now Donna's program is available to everyone and her promise to you is that if you take the knowledge in this book and use it in the way that she inspires you to, then you will have a better body in every conceivable way.

'This book is the next best thing to a clone of Donna in your handbag!'
–Brigitte Duclos, media personality

DONNA ASTON

FAT
OR FICTION

ARE YOU LIVING A FAIRY TALE?

Published by Hybrid Publishers

Melbourne Victoria Australia

© Donna Aston

This publication is copyright. Apart from any use as permitted under the Copyright Act 1968, no part may be reproduced by any process without prior written permission from the publisher. Requests and inquiries concerning reproduction should be addressed to the Publisher, Hybrid Publishers, PO Box 52, Ormond 3204.

First published 1999
Reprinted 1999
Reprinted with corrections 2000

National Library of Australia Cataloguing-in-Publication data:

Aston, Donna.
Fat or fiction: Are you living a fairy tale?

ISBN 1 876462 09 4.

1. Dietetics. 2. Body size. 3. Weight loss. I. Title.

613.2

Editor: Linda Roach
Photography: Christian Wild
Cover design: Scooter Design
Illustrations: Matt Golding

CONTENTS

ACKNOWLEDGMENTS

To my husband, Adrian, whom I adore, thank you for your patience, support and inspiration during the process of creating this book.

Thank you to Linda Roach, my editor, for her incredible dedication, talent and creativity. Louis de Vries, my publisher, thank you for believing in me and creating the high standard of publication we can now all enjoy reading.

Thanks to my training partner and best friend, Barry, for putting up with me through the gruelling Ms Universe competition preparations.

George Tabban at Muscle & Bodyshape Gymnasium, thank you for motivating me, 'kicking my butt', and helping me to create a body capable of representing Australia at the Ms Universe Figure Championships, 1999.

Finally, I'd like to thank all the people who have generously offered to share their experiences with us in this book.

DIE OLD ... STAY PRETTY

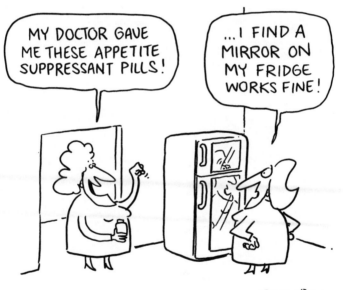

MY JOURNEY TO
FAT OR FICTION

Being an average teenager, you can imagine the horror of turning 18 and suddenly finding myself growing out instead of up! I gained weight at a steady rate over the next couple of years, reaching a grand peak of 80 kilograms at the age of 20! At this stage I considered myself to be around 20 kilograms over my ideal weight. This may not sound like an enormous gain to some, however, for me it was a nightmare come true! I became very depressed when my clothes would no longer fit and my once slim thighs were now bulging saddle-bags with 'cellulite' cascading down the back. I became a master of disguise, buying clothing with ample fabric to drape over my expanded rear-end. I needed help ... and fast!

Most men with a desire to lose weight will turn to exercise, whereas women usually rely on diet. I guess it has something to do with our early socialisation. Boys seem to be more involved in sports and physical activities than girls (although this seems to be changing) and so men's memories of being slim are probably associated with their days of playing football or other active sports. Women's emphasis on the food side of things has been swooped upon by the advertising industry and the media, only reinforcing this emphasis. Women's magazines bombard us with the latest, greatest ways to stop putting food in our mouths – you know the kind: 'The Food-Blending Diet' which shows you how to blend chicken and drink it through a straw so that you are exhausted before you've consumed enough to keep a chihuahua alive (at least you have burned off a few calories with all that sucking)!

I did what most women dieters have done. I resorted to attempts at severe calorie restriction, only to find my willpower wavering after a week or two and the weight returning in world-record time! This process was torture, both mentally and physically.

At the age of 21, after a full year of battling with calorie restriction in every way known to man (or should I say woman), I finally joined my local gym. I had tried other gyms in the past, only to find my attention span and motivation diminishing after two or three months. Frankly, I found the whole ordeal quite boring and I never seemed to achieve the desired result anyway. But I was ready to try again. The new gym I had chosen was one of those serious bodybuilding places – very intimidating to the novice trainer.

During three months of training correctly with the help of some of the 'serious' training guys at Mikes Gym, much to my amazement, my body began to change. At this point, I realised that I was capable of sculpting my body into any shape I desired, and so began an exciting journey to discover how to exercise and eat to make my body as healthy and fit and aesthetically pleasing as I could. If I was willing to make a concerted effort to learn more about how my body functioned, the sky was the limit! This became quite a personal challenge that has kept me learning and experimenting for more than ten years.

Just two years after I began training, I competed in a 'bodyshaping' competition weighing in at 55 kilograms and 8% body fat! This was an astounding loss of body fat when you consider that two years earlier I weighed around 80 kilograms with 35% body fat.

During ten years of competing, I won an Australian national competition, qualifying me to become the first Australian to earn professional status in my sport. I competed in the inaugural International Federation of Body Builders (IFBB) Ms Olympia Fitness Competition in 1995, in the bodyshaping section. Just a year later I placed eleventh in the IFBB World Professional Fitness Competition in New York. I was hooked!

I remain fascinated by the extraordinary physical condition that bodybuilders are capable of achieving. Bodybuilding – like it or hate it – is an amazing extreme of total physical and psychological conditioning. These athletes are indeed extremists, however there is a lot to be learned from their nutrition and training methods.

I am not suggesting that you should have such an extreme goal for yourself, however, I am saying that it is possible for anyone to reach his or her personal goals when armed with the appropriate knowledge and desire.

The first thing I had to learn when preparing for a competition was to focus on my body composition, as opposed to my weight on the scales. My goal was to lose only body fat, and at the same time, preserve muscle tissue. Now, this was tricky. If you eat too much food or the wrong kind of calories, you gain fat or do not lose it. If you eat too little food you lose muscle and fat, becoming thin but not lean. Yes, there is a huge difference.

I endured much trial and error before I perfected the technique to achieve my goal. At this time, I began to encounter an influx of people at the gym who desperately wanted my help. They had seen my achievements and wanted to know my 'secret'. Unfortunately, most people thought I had discovered a *magic carpet* and they wanted to climb aboard for a nice, easy ride!

When I told people that it took concentrated effort and discipline to reach this extreme physical conditioning, do you think that is what they wanted to hear? You guessed it!

I was all too aware, however, that all the effort and discipline in the world wouldn't be truly effective in the long term without the best information and methods; without the right stuff!

So began some serious research on this fascinating subject, in a quest to develop a system that worked for everyone, that could be easily tailored to fit the average person's lifestyle and that would enhance general health and wellbeing. I travelled to America in 1993 to meet with some medical professionals who had been researching the human body's metabolism and energy systems in relation to fat loss. I have studied a large number of medical research journals over the past 10 years and have written many articles on the subject of health and fitness for various Australian magazines. Readers of *Fitness Australia* magazine would know of the fitness challenges that I have conducted, one of which was with Brigitte Duclos, one of Australia's own television and radio celebrities. Brigitte's success was among my most positive results.

My personal experience and achievements; my core of knowledge gleaned from my search for 'the truth'; and my extensive career as a personal trainer have come together in this book. I am proud of it and believe that it can help you if you want it to.

I hope you enjoy reading this book as much as I have enjoyed writing it!

INTRODUCTION

The general aim of this book is to give you the knowledge to understand your body and its unique functions. With knowledge comes power: The power to *take control* of your body – its shape, its weight and its health – now and forever.

The number of diet and weight-loss alternatives available today is astounding. Statistically, almost half of the Australian population, both men and women, are in the 'obese' category! Every time we pick up a new magazine, we are bombarded with the *'latest craze'* in how to magically melt away the fat! Needless to say most are trying to *sell* us a new product. Each new and amazing system has the video, the audio-cassette, the book, the pill, the recipes, the shopping guide, the prepackaged foods ... and, don't forget, if you dial 1-800 immediately you'll receive a free set of steak knives!

Feeling confused and desperate to find the quickest and easiest method, of course we succumb. The diet industry makes millions of dollars telling us what we want to hear.

Have you ever noticed that with each new *gismo* on the market, comes the promise of not only fabulous results but fabulous results *faster*? We live in a society that craves instant gratification. Marketing gurus know that we want maximum results from minimum time and effort. Deep down inside, I think we actually know the truth. But we pick up the phone and give our credit card number ... just in case!

I am fascinated by so many of these publications and products. Many of them actually make claims that are physiologically incorrect, or impossible to achieve.

Now you need no longer follow these diet and exercise evangelists in a dozen different directions, chasing your tail!

The evolution of dieting insanity

The following list offers some insight into some of the crazy ideas dreamed up over a century (from where else but America!)

Year	Latest craze
1898	Horace Fletcher introduces his method of chewing food at a rate of 100 times per minute, having slimmed down from 205 pounds to 163 pounds.
1929	Advertisements for cigarettes, urging people to 'reach for a 'Lucky' (a cigarette brand) instead of a sweet – it's better for your figure!'
1930	The Hollywood Diet is all the rage. Eighteen days at 585 calories per day consisting of grapefruit, green vegetables, hard-boiled eggs and Melba toast.
1948	Two-thirds of patients treated for obesity are prescribed amphetamines, despite mounting evidence of their dangerous side-effects.
1981	The six-week, BeverleyHills Diet emerges, including 10 days of nothing but fruit!
1996	In a study of 2, 379 preadolescent girls, the American National Heart, Lung and Blood Institute finds that 40% of 9- and 10-year-olds were trying to lose weight.
1996	Approximately six million Americans are taking fen-phen, fenfluramine and phentermine (appetite suppressant and amphetamine), based on a 1992 study of their effectiveness. The products were pulled off the market by the FDA in 1997 (who had previously approved the drugs) due to side-effects of potentially fatal heart defects.
1998	The year of magic pills and plastic surgery, herbal cellulite 'cures', fat absorption medication, and a procedure called mega-liposuction!

In the year 2010, will our current methods of low-fat dieting be next on the list of dieting insanity?

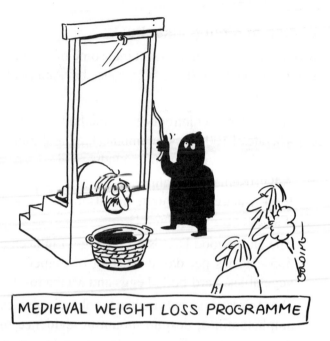

MEDIEVAL WEIGHT LOSS PROGRAMME

Knowledge is the key!

One of my clients once said to me, 'Donna, I just don't know what to believe. You answer my questions today, yet tomorrow I will pick up a fitness magazine and read something completely different. I don't even know what to eat for breakfast anymore!'

My answer to this commonly expressed dilemma is knowledge. Not biased, persuasive information but scientific facts about our bodies and how they function that can't be refuted or manipulated. This gentleman happened to be a very intelligent and successful businessman. I asked him whether he would have the same reaction if he were contradicted on a decision to buy a property, which he had investigated thoroughly and considered to be a sound investment. Would he jump up and down, not knowing what to do next, or would he use his understanding and knowledge to make an informed decision?

Of course, he chose the latter. This is *my* approach to nutrition and exercise. I have a complete understanding of *how* my body functions and *why* I do the things I do. I do not act on *hearsay*, even if the source of information seems reliable. I am open-minded enough to investigate new findings and ideas, however, my basic knowledge allows me to make calculated, informed decisions.

1
WHY THIS PROGRAM IS 'THE RIGHT STUFF'

The 'secret' to weight control

If you continue to follow the *same* strategy and apply yourself with the *same* amount of effort, you will be guaranteed to always achieve the s*ame* results! Whether this is used as a positive or a negative, it will always apply!

Let's look at some of the factors influencing our weight:

- Calories. We put on weight if we consume more calories than we burn off.
- Our Basal Metabolic Rate (BMR). This is the rate at which we burn calories and is determined by lean weight (muscle), genetics, hormones and exercise/activity levels.
- The nutritional value of the foods we consume – obtaining essential nutrients from food sources and manipulating ratios of macronutrients (protein, carbohydrates and fats) to meet the body's needs.

It's time we learned some basic facts! Many of us need to make some serious changes to our body image perspective if we have a desire to 'shape-up'. Observing our culture, it's only too obvious that we're obsessed with fat! The percentage of overweight individuals in the world is escalating into epidemic proportions. Most of us are far more focused on looking great in that new pair of skin-tight Levi's next weekend, than we are on our health. After all, we can't see all that stuff that's going on inside, so it's very easy to ignore. Unfortunately, 'all that stuff' on the inside will eventually make itself known to you, either through a general health decline, poor skin, hair and nails, lethargy, obesity, diabetes, high cholesterol levels, or countless other signs of an unhappy body. To aspire to look your best is admirable, however, it would not have been worth writing this book solely for that purpose. I think we are all aware that carrying around too much body fat is not just an issue of appearance and aesthetics, but may also be detrimental to our health.

Many people, in particular women, believe that you can never be too thin, going to great lengths to achieve 'the look'. This often leads to lowered metabolic rates and some very hungry, unsatisfied people. When it all gets too much to bear and the willpower dwindles, we severely reprimand ourselves for yet another failure, plunging our self-esteem to the ground.

You will probably agree that it is highly unlikely that you can solve a problem unless you know the cause.

There are a number of factors influencing why an individual puts on weight.

Everything you've read, every program you've joined, is the same old, repackaged version of a program that depends on some variation of calorie cutting – special plans to help you *eat less*! Whether they are tagged food combining, low-fat, or chewing your food while standing on your head, if you sit down and do your maths they will all add up to one thing – *calorie restriction.* Perhaps some of us do consume too many calories for the amount of activity we pursue, however, cutting calories alone is not the answer. Sure, you may see an initial drastic weight loss on the bathroom scales, but considering that 1 kilogram of fat is equivalent to 7, 700 calories, do you still think it is possible to lose 10 pounds of *fat* in 10 days? If this volume of weight loss is shown on the scales, it is almost certain to include a large percentage of both water and muscle tissue … not fat!

To prove to you that *their* system works, these programs must get results, fast! Remember, they are telling you what you *want* to believe, right?

Some of the latest statistics in Australia indicate a whopping $500 million dollars is spent annually on weight-loss products alone.

Americans spent a frightening $18 billion in 1996 on low-fat food products, $32 billion on weight-loss in general, and $45.8 billion on medical complications relating to obesity … Whoops! The cost of diet-related disease and obesity in 1988-89 was estimated at $672 million, with obesity-related, coronary heart disease and hypertension (high blood pressure) accounting for 62% of that amount. The cost of treating obesity within the healthcare system was $393 million! Statistically, a person is considered obese when his or her body weight is measured at more than 20% above his or her *ideal* weight.

The Consumer Advocacy and Financial Counselling Association of Victoria estimates that approximately 300,000 people purchase commercial weight-control programs each year at a cost of $500 million. The additional cost of anorectic agents, most of which do not fall within the Pharmaceutical Benefits Scheme, could be as high as $18 million a year. This estimate is based on the 410,000 prescriptions filled for such agents in 1989-90 at an average cost of $45 per prescription.

If you are willing to open your mind and allow me to tell you a little about how and why people are failing to achieve the bodies that they so desperately want, you may be pleasantly surprised to find that it all doesn't have to be that hard! In fact, like many things in life, *when you know how, it's downright easy!*

How do you know that this program will work any better than the others?

I've transformed myself from a pudgy, 80 kilogram girl, to a professional athlete training for international bodyshaping titles. I'm proof that my program works and, even more importantly, keeps working. Anyone can get results from this program.

Why? *Because you will never feel deprived and are free to enjoy 'real' food.*

This book contains practical advice for women and men from all walks of life, from the overweight businessman, to the 'fat conscious' teenage girl. The most common response from people has been one of relief. You will realise just how simple and logical it can be to improve your health, wellbeing and appearance. My intention is to revolutionise how to lose fat whilst maintaining optimum health. I intend to educate you on how to sustain a nutritionally balanced 'never-hungry' attitude towards food, with very little time commitment, or inconvenience.

There are enough diet books and weight-loss methods to resink the Titanic, but at what price? Some of these 'foolproof' methods could cost you your health and mental wellbeing as well as burning a huge hole in your pocket!

I have compared my program with many of the popular diet books on the market today. So far, not one of them compares to the superior nutritional values espoused in this book, which is based on 'real food' – getting back to basics! The so-called experts in recent years have complicated the approach to weight loss. Many people don't know what to believe anymore. This book will explain the concept of body composition and losing *fat*, as opposed to losing *weight*. This tones and shapes our body, as well as improving our general state of health. I've combined factual, scientific data with a 'headache-free' program. This will provide you with a user-friendly, reference manual designed to last you and your body a lifetime!

A testimonial from Hilary Willowsmith

At my age (fiftyish) I really started to become concerned about my health. I knew that many problems that women of my age face, such as osteoporosis and weight gain, could be avoided with regular exercise. I was never one to exercise but my husband had been working out with a personal trainer for a few months and getting great results. He was so enthusiastic about Donna that I decided to see her about starting a diet and exercise program.

I've always been a 'dieter'. At that stage I had an 'hourglass' figure – a smallish waist with lots of extra padding around the hips. I had spent almost an entire lifetime starving myself and then bingeing when it all became too hard.

At our first meeting I very proudly told Donna that I knew that low fat was the way to go but I just couldn't stick with it. At 65 kilograms with 38% body fat, appearances aside, I was well above the 'healthy' range.

I had never considered controlling sugars and carbohydrates in my previous diets and I often felt lethargic and bloated after meals, with a poor night's sleep to follow. After a relatively short time the dietary changes and exercise program that Donna instigated, made me not only look better, but feel better. I was finally in control!

I learned more with each passing week about my body. Donna taught me how to listen to its needs – how to recognise hunger, thirst, reactions to different foods and the need for rest and recovery.

I can now eat a larger volume of food and feel satisfied, never bloated or over-full. Because I eat 'real' food, whether I'm eating out with friends at a restaurant, or grabbing a bite to eat at work, it couldn't be easier or more socially acceptable. Most importantly of all, I've had no trouble staying on track; if anything, the more I learn and experience, built on Donna's foundation, the more motivated I become to keep this body forever! Now, almost four years later, I weigh 56 kilograms and have only 16.5% body fat! Instead of accepting the deterioration most people experience with ageing, I feel as if I am getting younger, fitter and healthier every year!

Hilary Willowsmith is a haute couturier and owner of Mortisha's Gothic clothing boutique in Melbourne

Hilary's statistics

1996	*1999*
Weight: 65 kg	Weight: 56 kg (9 kg loss)
Lean weight:40.06 kg	Lean weight: 44.64 kg (+4.58 kg)
Fat weight: 24.94 kg	Fat weight: 11.36 kg (-13.58 kg)
BMR: 1249 cals per day	BMR: 1455 cals per day

2
ARE YOU TOO FAT?

Reality bites!

Although most people talk about losing weight, if they realised that they were also losing muscles, bones and vital organ tissues (lean body weight), they would or should be horrified! We want to lose body fat alone!

The term *body composition* refers to what your body weight is composed of – stored fat and lean mass, ie, everything other than fat …muscle, internal organs, bones, etc.

The question, 'Are you too fat?', is not related to whether you can fit into size-8 jeans, or whether you fit the pigeon hole of the *correct height-to-weight* scale. 'Too fat' should refer to the fat percentage of your body weight. A healthy level for men is around 15%. For women, a level between 18 and 28% is considered healthy.

What relevance does this have to weight control? A lot more than you probably realise. We have been educated to pay attention to our total body weight – period. How many people do you know who *don't* have a set of bathroom scales? And I'll bet that most people (particularly women) give their scales a thorough workout!

Many government statistics and measurement charts are based on the height-to-weight scale for small-, medium- and large-framed individuals. How much you weigh is somewhat irrelevant to your body's health, tone, shape and appearance, due to one important, overlooked factor … body composition!

On most of these charts, many athletes would be falsely placed in the obese category due to their higher than normal lean-to-fat ratio which makes them heavier on the scales.

Whether your goal is to lose fat, tone muscle, gain more muscle size or become smaller, firstly we must have a method of measuring your current body composition in order to set realistic goals to change and monitor your progress. This can be simply and quickly achieved with an ultra-sound device or a skin-fold calliper test combined with statistics such as weight, height, age and sex. Most reputable gymnasiums and sports medicine clinics could advise you on this procedure. From this you can determine your personal calorie requirements and project the changes you wish to pursue.

I have seen many men and women who could only be described as skinny. They usually do not wish to lose weight, but to tone up. The fascinating thing about body composition is that even if a person appears to be very thin, he or she can still have a relatively high level of body fat, therefore appearing emaciated, yet soft and flabby at the same time. The reason for this is a low level of lean tissue and a higher level of stored body fat. To 'tone up', he or she should basically follow the same program as a person who is overweight, in order to reduce body fat and gain lean tissue. This is the definition of tone – high lean mass and low body fat. For women to appear 'toned and firm', they would probably need to achieve a body composition with around 18%-20% fat. This is lower than that of the average woman, yet still considered within the healthy range. Unfortunately, the lack of awareness or understanding of these facts often leads to the development of eating disorders and body-image distortions in many teenagers. They attempt to lose weight on the scales without realising that their real desire is to change their body composition, or 'tighten and tone'!

Obviously aesthetic considerations should not be the sole reason for improving our body composition. Health and wellbeing should be high on our priority list. By maintaining a body composition in a healthy range, we can eliminate the risk of many debilitating ailments, diseases and stresses that our body may endure if we are over-fat.

How you dress your skeleton is up to you!

Imagine identical twins of the same height and structure. We will call them Anne and Maree. They jump on the bathroom scales and they both weigh 60 kg. But Maree is always complaining that Anne can eat whatever she likes without putting on weight, whereas she may as well just bypass her mouth and stick the cake to her hips because that's where it is going anyway! Maree believes that Anne is just lucky. What she doesn't realise is that her sister has only 20% body fat while she has 40%. So who burns more calories?

Anne	**Maree**
60 kg	60 kg
20% body fat	40% body fat
48 kg lean weight	36 kg lean weight
12 kg fat weight	24 kg fat weight
Basal Metabolic Rate (BMR)	BMR
approx. 1500 calories per day	approx. 1000 calories per day

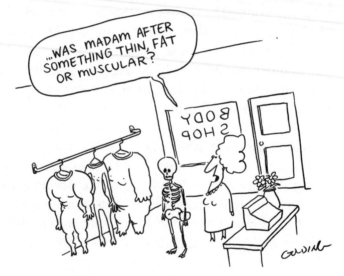

- The term basal metabolic rate refers to the amount of calories the body uses in a state of complete rest (without activity) to keep us alive.
- A calorie is actually a unit of measurement used to indicate the energy value of foods.

Even when completely rested, the body must be burning calories at a steady rate to perform vital functions, such as repair and cell replacement, organ functions and core temperature maintenance. The BMR is determined largely by the lean weight of an individual, along with the influences of hormones, genetics and activity levels. The higher your lean weight, the larger your body's engine or furnace, the more fuel it will burn. Therefore, more calories can be consumed before an excess is stored in the form of body fat.

An effective analogy would be to compare a large car with a V8 engine, with a small 4-cylinder car. If you monitor the petrol gauge, which one would burn the most fuel, even whilst idling? Obviously the larger engine.

As a rough estimate, for every kilogram of lean muscle tissue you gain, you will burn approximately 50 *extra* calories at rest, every day! Unfortunately, this works both ways. For every kilogram of lean muscle tissue you lose, whether through lack of essential nutrients or lack of physical activity, you will burn approximately 50 calories *less* per day. You can now see that a 'low metabolic rate', which is commonly used as an excuse for being over-fat, is far more in your control than first thought.

The 'ideal' healthy female has statistically around 24% body fat, however, many women have well in excess of 35%. Usually only elite female athletes are measured at below 15% body fat.

The 'ideal' healthy male has statistically around 15% body fat, however, it is not unusual for inactive men to measure at well over 30% body fat. Elite male athletes may measure at as low as 4% body fat.

Anyway, to get back to our twins. Maree decides that she wants to lose weight so she restricts her calorie intake to 900 per day. Her body doesn't know that she is intentionally depriving it of food – she could be starving to death in the middle of the Sahara Desert. If she sustains this 'willpower' for long enough, her body will automatically move into survival mode. One of the body's strongest inbuilt mechanisms is to try to sustain life at all costs. During times of famine the body will become as energy efficient as it has to. So what does it discard first? Expendable lean tissue. This will create a smaller furnace, therefore lowering the body's BMR and hence its calorie requirements.

After a month or two on this diet, Maree, like the overwhelming majority of dieters, quits. It is just too hard to maintain so she returns to her previous way of eating. But now she has lost valuable lean muscle tissue and no longer needs as many calories as before.

She will now store excess fat even faster and she won't know why. She will eventually diet again and the yo-yo cycle will continue.

After the age of 20, those who do not do regular weight training exercise lose an average of 250 grams of muscle tissue per year.

Genetic traits – blessings or curses?

The body has tissue located on the back of the neck known as 'brown fat'. The brown coloration is due to a high concentration of fat-burning units called mitochondria. This fat produces energy for heat production, as opposed to energy for movement, enabling us to adapt to cold weather. It is thought that the brain can stimulate brown fat to produce heat when excess food is consumed, to control weight gain. Due to our predetermined genetic traits, some people may have insufficient amounts of brown fat, or a faulty message pathway from the brain to signal effective usage. This may be yet another factor influencing our metabolic system.

Are you an apple or a pear?

Most people could describe their fat distribution and thus their body shape as resembling a pear or an apple. In other words, a majority of fat is accumulated either on the upper (apple) or lower (pear) section of the body.

Upper body and abdominal obesity can be quite detrimental to our health, due to the fact that it is often primarily *visceral fat* (within the abdominal cavity). This type of fat is more metabolically active and is much easier to shed than subcutaneous fat (beneath the skin), however, an excess surrounds the internal organs creating a strain on their functions. Abdominal fat drains directly to the liver, and can interfere with HDL (good cholesterol) production.

Subcutaneous fat (directly beneath the skin), which makes up much of the fat on the hips, bottom and thighs does not carry as great a health risk, if any at all. Different concentrations of each type of fat vary amongst individuals. The volume stored of both fats is obviously determined by our lifestyle, however, the ratio of the fats is predetermined by our genetics. The stored fat in women's thighs fulfils the biological function of a reserve energy supply in the case of famine during pregnancy. This is why many underweight, malnourished women's menstrual cycles cease when body fat drops *too low*.

Our hypothetical twins may both weigh 60 kilograms, however, due to the difference in body composition, we really have a 48 kilogram person carrying around 12 kilograms of stored fat and a 36 kilogram person carrying 24 kilograms of stored fat.

No wonder Anne can consume more food (therefore nutrients), without storing any excess energy in the form of body fat.

If it were possible to change your body composition to the obviously preferred, leaner option, wouldn't you like to commit yourself to achieving it?

If the answer is, 'Yes' … then read on!

A testimonial from Roland Rocchiccioli

Exercise can be very boring! It takes real determination and long-term commitment to drag yourself off to the gymnasium and put yourself through the paces. It is so easy to lose interest when you fail to see immediate results. An over-indulgence in cakes and puddings had thickened my waist. It came time for some hard work if I was to appear on television, on Channel Nine's 'The Footy Show', and stand alongside some of the nation's fittest athletes.

I first met Donna Aston at Colt's Gym and, for me, it proved to be a fantastic meeting. Having worked with her on several occasions I have to conclude that she knows more about exercise, food and getting results, than anyone I have ever met. Donna has the rare and incredible capacity to keep you interested in your own progress; she is a constant source of encouragement when you feel that nothing is happening; and, most importantly, she varies the program to keep you interested.

Donna speaks such good sense! She not only has the knowledge but great ability to impart it. I remember when she first spoke to me about her book. I was certain it was a wonderful concept and later, when I saw several of the completed chapters, I knew!

I have always wanted to use the wonderfully old-fashioned phrase: 'I have no hesitation in recommending her to anyone who might require her services.' If you are serious about your food and exercise program, this is the book for you.

Donna will change your life.

Roland Rocchiccioli is a media personality and author.

3
A LOOK AT EATING DISORDERS ...

... Why have they become so prevalent in our society?

In the past, and still today in some societies, fat was seen as a very desirable asset. In cultures where the mark of the peasant, who toiled all day and had little to eat, was leaness, fat was prized as a sign of wealth.

Today, in our society, where food is plentiful and being fat is easy, slimness is the goal — a sign of beauty and self-control. Women grow up believing that to be attractive; to get the 'look', they must be thin. Under this intense pressure 'normal' women often become obsessive about weight control to the point where it dominates their lives.

Obviously, along the continuum of eating disorders there are those who have deeper psychological issues and who need a great deal of support in that area. I do believe, however, that there are many women who get caught up in destructive eating patterns because they do not have the knowledge and understanding to achieve success with their bodies; the knowledge to create healthier, firmer, leaner bodies.

Instead they focus their attention on the scales in that continual quest to weigh less. Thus the spiral into disordered eating. They eat less and less or they eat uncontrollably and regurgitate. Often, excessive exercising accompanies the eating problem.

During the twelve years that I have been working in the health and fitness area I have come across many people, mainly young women, who have had some degree of eating disorder. The majority of them are, sadly, just setting themselves up to become fatter and fatter. Some do become excessively thin and reach a nice low number on the scale. Are they then happy with their new bodies? Of course not. By starving themselves, they have lost mostly lean tissue and therefore their muscles become flaccid, their skin becomes loose, and the 'look' is not achieved. And they are probably seriously compromising their health.

It is quite amazing to observe the attempts our bodies make to protect life when threatened with starvation. Your body doesn't know that you are deliberately abstaining from food and will assume that it is a time of famine. In reaction to this, the menstrual cycle often ceases (amenorrhoea), indicating that your body is in no state to bear a child, seeing as you are struggling to sustain your own life. Another protective mechanism is the growth of fine, downy, usually blond hair all over the body. This is the body's way of trying to insulate you against the elements, as your layer of fat beneath the skin normally would.

Anorexia nervosa

I am going to share with you a true story of someone dealing with anorexia nervosa.

As a ballet dancer, it was not unusual for Susan to appear emaciated and sinewy in her structure. At first she seemed to be in self-denial concerning her problem, but as I got to know her a little better, we began to discuss diet and exercise. These conversations allowed me to understand how Susan's battle with weight had begun and what factors perpetuated it. It is common, indeed even prerequisite, for ballet dancers to be abnormally thin in order to portray the dance in an elegant and delicate way. But the effects of Susan's self-induced starvation and abuse of her body were quite prominent and went way beyond the norm for dancers.

Her prematurely aged skin, her thin, lifeless hair, brittle fingernails and, perhaps the turning point for Susan herself, the body density of an 80-year-old woman!

Susan confessed to drinking Diet Coke when she felt hungry because the bubbles made her stomach feel full. Occasionally, she would have a 'Cup of Soup' for lunch, or just a coffee. I remember being horrified when she shared stories with me about some of the other dancers she worked with. They would make comparisons with one another to see who could count the most visible ribs in their sternum (breast bone). It was considered desirable to boast the most visible bones!

Susan agreed to work with me to try and prevent any further wasting of her bone structure and to improve her health. A convincing factor for her was that I weighed a considerable amount more than she, yet we had the same percentage of body fat. For Susan this was an entirely new concept. Susan was around 170 cm (5'7") tall and weighed a mere 42 kilograms, with 10% body fat. At only 3 cm taller, I weighed 60 kilograms and yet had the same percentage of body fat. Obviously her loss of bone density and severe muscle wasting contributed to such a light total weight. My aim was to teach her that she could eat a healthy quantity of food, gain weight on the scales, yet still remain at 10% body fat. The scales had always been her method of measurement; sometimes she weighed herself 10 times a day. She would weigh herself after she ate or drank, after she exercised or at any time of the day that she 'felt fat'!

I agreed to test her body-fat level with an ultrasound device. This is the most accurate simple way of measuring body fat. Of course, if you have access to an under-water hydrostatic tank (available at some universities and sports institutes) or a laboratory that has 'dual electron x-ray absorptiometry' you could get an absolutely accurate reading of body fat! I promised to test Susan's body-fat level everyday, even twice a day if she felt it was necessary. She agreed to disregard what she was seeing on the scales and use the body-fat measurement as our guide. There were many habits to break and many psychological obstacles to overcome. The intensity of fear Susan felt seeing those scales jump up even half a kilogram was astounding; she could only be consoled with the 'proof' of an ultrasound test indicating lean gain, no fat!

This process took several months to establish, eventually proving to Susan that she could gain weight on the scales, yet not get any fatter. I have found that the fear of most people is that if they weigh more then they are bigger and fatter. They associate fat with the bathroom scales. The immediate assumption is that the less we weigh, the leaner, more toned and slimmer we will appear … right?

... wrong! This is where we need education about body composition!

I have heard stories, often described as horrific by anorexic women, about the medical profession's solution to the problem. The 'solution' most disturbing to many sufferers is hospitalisation, where they are basically force fed intravenously until they reach their 'correct' weight. Obviously, lying in a bed and being fed in this way encourages a weight gain of fat alone, not lean tissue. Women would be released from the hospital, only to feel *totally disgusted* with their fatter, 'healthier' bodies and would return to their old habits. Thus their belief that an increase in weight means an increase in fat would be confirmed!

Susan went through all sorts of dilemmas with her exercise and eating habits. During an exercise session in the gym, I turned her body to face a mirror to explain the movement of an exercise, only to see tears begin to stream down her cheeks. At first, I thought she had hurt herself. When I asked her what was wrong, she sobbed, 'I can't stand to look at my ugly body in the mirror'. On another occasion I had made some 'protein cream' (see recipe section). Susan asked to try some, so I gave her a bit on the end of a teaspoon. When she asked what was in it and my response was 'cream', she actually spat it out, running into the bathroom to wash her mouth out. Just the thought of eating something that contained calories made her gag!

I am very pleased to say, that today, three years later, Susan weighs a stable and lean 57 kilograms, with a bone density measurement at the lower end of the 'normal' range. At least it is now *in the range*. She also maintains a very low 10-12% body fat, at which she feels comfortable. Obviously this is still a very low body-fat level to maintain, however, she is now stabilising it within her comfort zone in a healthy manner, using my program of sensible exercise and diet. I am pleased to say that Susan eats like a horse!

Bulimia (binge and purge syndrome)
This may sound like the opposite problem to anorexia, however, it is very closely related. The development of this disorder seems to always be associated with psychological aspects, often leading

sufferers to believe that they are 'abnormal', further lowering their self-esteem. I believe there are sometimes 'lifestyle' reasons or physical circumstances that can be dealt with on a much simpler level.

Bulimia describes the bingeing of foods, often sweets, followed immediately by self-induced vomiting, or use of laxatives to rid the body of the calories consumed. It is usually done secretly and is rarely admitted to or discussed by the sufferer.

One particular client comes to mind. When Elaine walked into my office, she explained that she felt overweight, had very low self-esteem and wanted to make some changes to her lifestyle. After visiting a reputable dietitian one week prior to our appointment, she was feeling rather disillusioned. She had poured her heart out to this 'expert' only to be given a booklet on *How to be fat and happy*, while being instructed not to be so *hung-up* on her body image. As I spoke to Elaine, she appeared to be very troubled by this 'problem'and believed that she needed some help to solve it. She had been made to feel that her problem was trivial however she was not only concerned about losing weight, but also about the effects of her 10 kilogram weight gain over the past three years on her health. We measured her body composition at 38% body fat. This was quite a bit higher than the healthy range of 18–28%. As she felt more comfortable speaking to me, Elaine also admitted having a binge/purge problem. She felt that this had developed as a result of frustration at gaining weight and losing control. Elaine would try to diet, restricting calories to ridiculously low levels for a few days. When her willpower gave out, she would binge on any food she could get her hands on, then, feeling guilty for being so 'weak', she would purge … and the cycle would begin again.

As I have explained earlier, if you cut calories below your basal metabolic requirement, your body will react with *urgent* physical cravings that will become very hard to resist. You can't succeed in 'tricking' your body in this way … its built-in survival mechanism is far too sophisticated for that!

As Elaine and I talked through the changes in her lifestyle over the period in which she had gained the weight, we established a number of obvious contributing factors including the commencement of a sedentary job, injuring her ankle and giving up walking to work. She began to understand that it was not some 'out of control' disease that had struck her, just a combination of gradual, unintentional changes which could be easily reversed. We started Elaine on a light exercise plan and 'cleaned up' her diet. With the knowledge she gained about her body and its reactions to her lifestyle, Elaine was able to take control and create the changes necessary to improve her health and lose the excess kilos.

There can be physical triggers involved in this disorder, for example, a reaction to health problems such as low blood sugar (hypoglycaemia), an unbalanced diet, too much refined carbohydrate and low levels of essential nutrients, hormonal imbalances, and food allergies and sensitivities. Usually sufferers will blame themselves for being weak and lacking willpower. The body will naturally *crave* foods if it is not fed the nutrition it needs. If blood sugar levels fluctuate more than they should (usually due to poor diet, or attempts at calorie restriction), the body will automatically crave sweet foods in an attempt to stabilise it. Our natural physical demands are not easy to ignore and should *not* be ignored. Instead, we need to learn why the craving is there in the first place and eliminate it from the source.

4
MOVE IT AND LOSE IT!

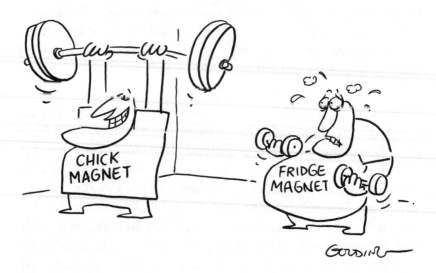

Together with our poor diets, our relatively sedentary lifestyle adds substantially to the weight-control dilemma. Although technology has freed us from many hours of drudgery, it has robbed us of the necessity to work our bodies. Although it has given us more time for leisure we seem to be leading more hectic, frenetic lives than ever before. This makes exercise even more imperative. But how could you possibly make time in your busy day to exercise? Well, before you answer, think about this:

Most women will gain an average of around 8 kilograms of body fat between the ages of 25 and 55. How many calories in excess (overeaten or not burned) per day do you think it would take for this to occur? *Believe it or not, as little as 5–10 calories per day!*

The 'secret' is, that in order to burn our stored body fat, and/or control our fat levels, *all* daily activity is beneficial! Yes, that's right! It all adds up.

Studies have shown that a minimum of just 50 extra calories burned per day can induce change. It does not matter what type of activity you do – just do it!

I would bet that some of you have never considered housework exercise. Gardening, playing with the children, walking the dog, washing the car, vacuuming … they all have a positive effect! Take the stairs instead of the elevator at work or park a little further away from the office and walk. The time commitment is minimal, if not nonexistent, when you incorporate activity into everyday tasks.

How do you know how many calories you are currently burning, or what your goal should be? There is a simple formula to give you an indication of the values of calories:

7,700 calories = 1 kilogram of stored body fat.

In other words, to gain or lose one kilogram of stored body fat, we must first tilt the energy balance equation 7,700 calories the appropriate way.

An adult would burn an average of approximately 300 calories in one hour of brisk walking. A McDonalds Big Mac has around 500 calories, a Mars chocolate bar has 300 calories. Get the picture?

For those of you who indulge in a large helping of Black Forest cake after dinner, with the intention of 'burning it off' with a brisk, 10-minute walk around the block in the morning, think again! In fact, a quick pace for around an hour and a half might just do it!

It is very easy to consume *empty,* concentrated calories, with the popularity of processed foods, but very difficult to burn them off. Be wary of weight-loss programs that claim to make you lose a large amount of weight in a short space of time. It is not possible to shed 'fat' at a *fast* rate. If a large quantity of weight is lost on the scales, you can guarantee that a large percentage of it is muscle and water … not fat! As with all fads, you will resume a normal eating pattern eventually and regain the lost weight, but this time in the form of excess body fat, not muscle, due to a lowered *basal metabolic rate.*

As a fitness consultant, I am constantly being asked, 'What is better for burning calories – walking or jogging?' or 'How long do I need to exercise for?' My answer to both questions is, '*Just move!*'

Don't complicate things, just believe that all activity is cumulative.

As you can now work out, the calories in one kilogram of body fat are equivalent to over 25 hours of walking for the average sized adult. I don't want to discourage you, but I think it is very important to have all of this information in perspective to enable you to reach realistic goals in a reasonable amount of time.

You can safely reduce your calorie intake without negative side effects if:

•   you are over-consuming calories to begin with
•   you do not reduce calories below your basal metabolic rate.
For example:

Jane's BMR is measured at 1200 calories per day. She is currently consuming 2000 calories, which is 800 over her BMR. Her daily activity burns an average 500 calories, which leaves her with 300 excess calories per day. If Jane reduced her food intake to 1600 calories per day (-400) and increased her activity to 600 per day (+100), she would be in debt of 200 calories per day, therefore encouraging safe fat loss. Jane's daily calorie intake should never drop below 1200, or she will risk losing lean tissue and becoming deficient in nutrients. This could cause a reduction in her metabolic rate and suppress her immune system, actually hindering her fat loss efforts and leaving her body susceptible to illness.

Following this regime, Jane could burn approximately one kilogram of body fat every 38 days. Of course, if she were to increase her rate of activity further, the results would occur much sooner.

Keep in mind that a loss of *stored body fat only* is a very noticeable one. One kilogram of *pure fat loss* can change your appearance significantly.

Imagine the diagram below is the petrol gauge in your car. If you were to fill your car with petrol above the 1800 calorie maintenance marker, there would be an excess or overflow of fuel. This also applies to Jane when she consumes more than 1800 calories per day with her activity level. She would therefore be consuming an excess of fuel/calories, leaving that remaining 'overflow' available for storage – commonly known as fat!

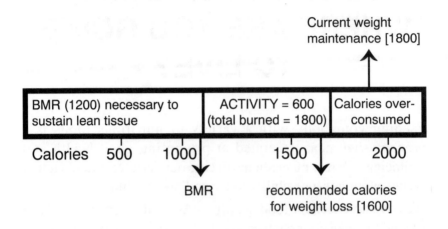

Fat is a lighter substance than densely constructed muscle tissue, yet it takes up a great deal more volume. If you are old enough to remember the old-fashioned milk bottles, before milk was homogenised, you will recall that the cream separated from the milk and floated on the top because the fat was lighter. When we lose *muscle tissue*, a greater quantity of weight loss is apparent on the scales, with little visible result. When we achieve *fat loss,* even one kilogram occupies a great deal of space, therefore showing a significant change in appearance, rather than just a lower reading on the scales.

5

IF YOU DON'T LOOK AFTER YOUR BODY, WHERE ARE YOU GOING TO LIVE?

Feeding your body with a variety of nutritious foods is a *preventative* measure aimed at promoting good health and wellbeing. We rely on medicine to cure our diseases, often without taking enough responsibility to try and prevent illness.

We have an excellent food supply in Australia, however most of us tend to make poor choices. Next time you go shopping, look at the contents of various shopping trolleys (perhaps your own should be included!). When you find them crammed with potato crisps, soft drinks, frozen party pies and sweet biscuits, you will probably see the effects of these poor food choices on the people pushing the trolleys!

At the turn of the century, food processing began to refine many essential nutrients, such as vitamins B6 and E, and the mineral magnesium from our food sources. At the same time, man-made fats, known as 'trans-fatty acids', were introduced and further hindered the nutrient value of our food. The heart attack epidemic began after 1920. Coincidental? I think not!

Food facts

- A survey conducted by the Australian Bureau of Statistics found that more than 20% of the energy intake of Australian children is derived from soft drinks, confectionery, biscuits, cakes, takeaway food and snack products.
- Recent surveys on nutrition show that up to 60% of the Australian population is deficient in one or more of the essential nutrients.

- Over 70% of women aged 25-55 years participating in the 1983 National Dietary Survey in Australia had iron intakes below the recommended daily intake.
- In a 1992 survey of 120 Australian children, 28% of those tested were iron deficient.
- Up to 90% of people have diet regimes deficient in Omega 3 fatty acids.
- 50% of hospital patients studied in the USA developed nutritional deficiencies eating hospital food!
- Less than 0.5% of the human population have 'bad genes' causing degenerative diseases, yet 68% of the population eventually die from degenerative diseases.

Many people look after a car more lovingly than their own body! You *know* that if you put inferior fuel in your car and don't service the engine, it will eventually break down. Most people would not keep driving their car until the doors fall off and the tyres rot, before they have the car attended to and yet they are prepared to neglect the maintenance of their bodies.

It is sad, but true that too many of us are more concerned with our *appearance* than our *health*. Knowing that this is true, I have focused much of this book on improving your physical appearance, with the underlying but essential bonus of improved health thrown in!

A testimonial from Barry Burd

At long last I have found the 'yellow-brick road' to more energy and less fat! I am 36 years old and had always found it difficult to control my weight. However, for the past three years I have managed to maintain my new physique. Maintenance is the key word for me.

For 22 years I have followed all the famous 'miracle' diets (and some not so well-known ones too!). Sure, on most of these diets I could lose weight but I usually felt hungry, tired and irritable, and I could never maintain the loss. The fat always returned, bringing with it some extra buddies, and so the jeans went up two sizes!

Then came Donna. Her approach to eating and exercise makes being healthy and staying lean achievable. She has given me so much knowledge about my body, and how and why it reacts to the changes I choose to make. What she says seems so simple and logical and yet most 'dieters' just don't know about it.

A fabulous side-effect of following Donna's program was a dramatic improvement in my skin. Having suffered from psoriasis and eczema for most of my life this was an unexpected bonus.

I believe that the changes I have made have had such a positive effect on the outside, that my body is much happier on the inside!

Barry Burd is a Melbourne hairdresser.

6
SO ... HOW SHOULD WE EAT?

The calories we consume are made up of three main components, each with its own specific function or purpose.

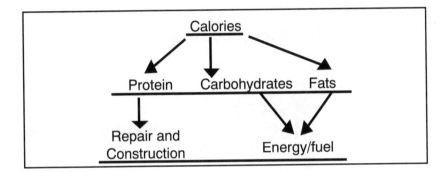

The above diagram indicates the basic components of calories and their purpose.

Protein is responsible for repair and construction of every cell in your body, including your hair, nails, muscle, blood, tendons and skin. Many health authorities recommend that we consume 10–15% of our daily calories in the form of protein, 65–75% in the form of carbohydrates, and as little fat as possible – approximately 10–20%.

Does it make sense to you that we only take in 10% of our total calories for the purposes of repair and construction of every cell in our bodies?

We are battling to keep our stored body fat down, yet we are advised to consume 90% of our calories in foods which are used by the body exclusively as fuel/energy, which in turn we must burn off everyday to avoid excess fat deposition!

The following diagrams show the very dated, traditional food pyramid recommended by most health and medical authorities and an updated version, adapted to accommodate our changing lifestyle, and food availability into the 21st century. This pyramid is designed to provide optimum nutrition and to maximise fat-burning potential.

As you can see, the *old* food pyramid does not use our newly-discovered knowledge about fats and oils to differentiate between those that are *essential* to our health and those that are *detrimental*. Surely we can't group essential fish oils – proven time and time again to have undisputed health benefits – with trans-fatty acids found in processed oils used for deep frying, margarine, etc.

The dietary food pyramid

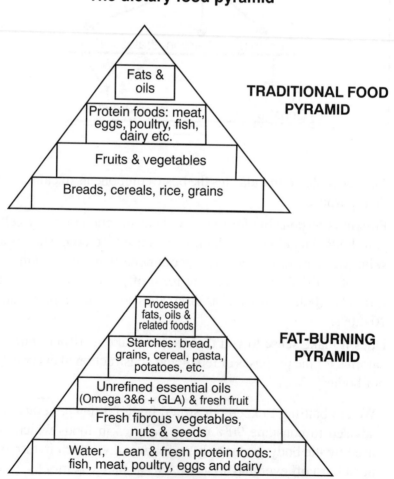

The traditional pyramid says that if it's fat, it must be bad!

People worldwide have been attempting to follow, even loosely, the traditional food pyramid for years now ... but we're getting fatter! I certainly subscribe to the addage, 'If it's not broken, don't fix it!' But it *is* broken and the very fact that you are reading this book shows that you may not be satisfied with the results you are currently achieving. Statistics show that our nation is getting fatter, and this fat is bringing with it all of the associated ill health – diabetes, chronic-fatigue syndrome, cancers, heart disease, immune deficiencies ... the list goes on and on.

When we consume an excessive amount of any calories, whether protein, carbohydrate or fat, it will be converted in the liver to storable fat and transported to the fat cells where it awaits the opportunity to be used.

Cutting fat from the diet will not automatically reduce fat stores in the body, even though it will have the biggest impact on calorie reduction, as discussed earlier. Of all our nutrients, processed carbohydrates are the most commonly over-consumed component in modern-day diets.

Remember that carbohydrates can be converted to fat for storage in the body if consumed to excess. Australia currently consumes 13.2% of its total calories in the form of sucrose (refined sugar) and an astounding 22.9% in the form of flour. (Australian Bureau of Statistics).

If you were to run a marathon everyday of your life you could probably eat as many fuel calories as your heart desired. Perhaps it would not be a particularly balanced diet, but you would probably have very little excess fat deposition. As this is highly unlikely for any of us, I would suggest it is logical to structure our food intake around our lifestyle to produce a happy, healthy body.

The caveman diet

Before agriculture and medicine our distant ancestors were hunter/ gatherers and they ate 'real' food. Of course they had no choice, there were no processed, no refined, no enriched, no manufactured foods. And they didn't get fat! I know; I know; they died young and they probably didn't look all that pretty, but the point I'm making is that if we can combine the elements of the caveman diet with the wonders of medicine and disease prevention, and our knowledge about creating optimum health for our minds as well as our bodies, we can't help but get it right.

If it was manmade ... don't eat it!

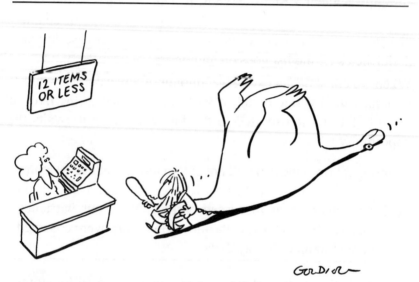

A testimonial from Emma McLean

Donna has advised and trained me over a period of about seven years and I have had great success following a sensible, balanced and achievable program of exercise and diet.

Donna is very dedicated and extremely well researched, and completely committed in her pursuit of physical health. The basis of her advice is good research and she is always prepared to refine and modify as she broadens her reference and contact base.

Donna has a wealth of experience and knowledge that translates into a successful program.

Emma McLean, Bachelor of Applied Science (Physical education), is a director of television production company, Prime Time Productions.

7
UNDERSTANDING DIETING METHODS AND FAT LOSS

Use your intellect and you won't need willpower!

How to detect a 'rip off' weight-loss plan

If a weight loss program prescribes a reduction in calories below your BMR together with:

- no exercise or physical effort or
- unrealistic promises of fast weight loss or
- sales of the latest cream, pill or potion,

you can be confident that it is a *scam!* Such 'magical' programs will not only disappoint you through lack of promised results, but they may also harm your health, not to mention burning a hole in your pocket.

Some side-effects of such programs may include:

- loss of lean tissue (predominantly muscle), causing your BMR to decrease. In short, this means that *fat gain* occurs when *normal* calorie intake is resumed (remember the twins) ... hence the so-called yo-yo syndrome
- loss of vital nutrition
- a lack of energy and endurance, which automatically reduces fat-burning activity.

Many commercial programs actually discourage exercise, particularly weight training. The reason behind this is that they teach you to measure your progress on the scales. They want you to see quick results, therefore, loss of muscle tissue is going to show a greater reduction in total body weight – very deceiving! If you were to retain your lean tissue (muscle) and lose only stored body fat, this would hinder *their* desired outcome on the scales!

Even if these *magic* diet plans do not appear to be focusing on calorie restriction, they usually are. Low-fat means low-calorie, plain and simple. Fat has the highest value of calories of all the nutrients we consume. One gram of fat has nine calories, one gram of protein or carbohydrate has four calories. You may automatically reduce your total calorie intake when you begin to eat the types of food that your body requires for optimal nourishment. When the body is satisfied with a balanced, daily intake of vitamins, minerals and all essential nutrients, your volume of food may be greater, however, the caloric value is quite often less and you lose food cravings. It is still important, however, not to drop below your basal metabolic requirement.

The human body is a remarkable machine. It will adapt and adjust its system to preserve life. It will continue to fine-tune all systems and functions as we try to trick and out-smart it. If your main focus is on the bathroom scales, you are probably quite proud of yourself for exhibiting the willpower to diligently adhere to your latest calorie restrictions.

As many of us have discovered, it takes incredible willpower to voluntarily sustain the feeling of hunger for prolonged periods of time. Restricting calories is like holding your breath ... when you begin to breathe again, you gasp for copious amounts of oxygen; after calorie deprivation you are desperate to feast!

With the lower metabolic rate you have created by losing valuable muscle tissue, that fat will be cascading down those thighs again in no time! I think that most of us, men and women alike, would like to reshape our bodies, as opposed to keeping the same shape and just getting a little smaller. If you do not focus your efforts on changing body composition, but instead on *weight loss*, at best, you will become a smaller version of the shape you are now and probably not permanently.

Generally, after several attempts at this spasmodic ritual, our bodies look and feel in worse shape than when we began! Perhaps this explains why *the latest research has proven that 95% of all weight-loss clinic clientele regain weight.*

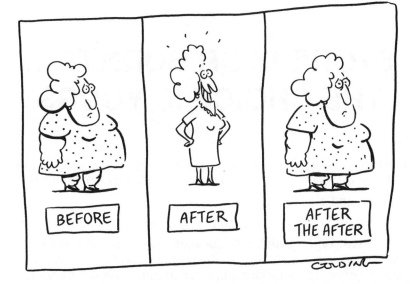

It is usually at this point that we begin to search for blame. Age is one reason I hear repeatedly. As we age we become less active, full stop! Picture a family get-together. What are the children doing and what are the adults doing? Well, I immediately see the image of adults lazing around the food area, eating, drinking and catching up on the latest gossip ... probably complaining about how they have just eaten *too much food*! The children, however, are running, playing and far too busy to even *think* about food, until their parents force them to sit still for long enough to eat something!

And, you must have heard this: 'It gets harder and harder to lose weight as you get older and, anyway, you are more susceptible to injuries if you exercise too much.'

Obviously, as we get older, we have more responsibilities, less time, perhaps a sedentary job, a vehicle to take us *everywhere* – excuses, excuses, excuses! We create these habits, so therefore it is completely within our power to make changes, at the very least, to modify our lifestyle, *without* great time commitments, to allow for a healthier and more active existence.

Changing the nutritional composition of your diet in ways that are compatible with your lifestyle, and increasing your daily activity and therefore the calories burned, combine to give you a sustainable, logical and healthy method of losing stored body fat ... forever!

8
STORE IT OR BURN IT ...
THE CHOICE IS YOURS

The often overlooked factor in the store it or burn it issue is your ability to manipulate two substances naturally secreted by the body – insulin and glucagon.

One of these is always dominant in your system, while the other is suppressed. Both insulin and glucagon play important roles.

Insulin encourages fat storage, whereas glucogon stimulates the fat burning process.

I think it is quite obvious which of the two we would like to remain dominant! Believe it or not, you are very capable of choosing which of the two *you* want to be in control! Of the three food components – protein, carbohydrates and fats – only one releases significant amounts of insulin when consumed – carbohydrates! The more *processed* the carbohydrate source, the sharper the surge of insulin release.

Our insulin levels rise when we eat carbohydrates, signalling to the body that we have an abundance of energy food in our system, therefore suppressing glucogon release because the body does not require any stored fat to be released as fuel. As soon as we modify our carbohydrate intake to consist mainly of fibrous vegetables, eliminating all refined sugars and flour products, we allow glucagon levels to rise, stimulating stored fat mobilisation as an energy source.

It is no coincidence that Type 2 diabetics receiving insulin injections struggle with weight gain. Most of the medical profession still refuses to acknowledge this insulin/obesity connection. Another side effect that Type 2 diabetics commonly suffer from, when taking insulin injections, is elevated cholesterol levels ... what a coincidence ... or is it?

Whether you are exercising in the gym, or just doing your daily chores, you will be allowing your body to access stored body-fat reserves for the purpose it was stored in the first place – energy!

How do you 'burn' fat?

You have probably been told 1,000 times by diet and exercise 'gurus' that you must sustain aerobic exercise for a minimum period of 20 minutes to dip into your fat reserves for fuel. If you eat a diet high in refined carbohydrates, then yes, your body will have no choice but to burn carbohydrates as its primary fuel source, at least until it uses up immediately available reserves (which, by the way, may take hours). When carbohydrate stores are finally exhausted, what do you think your body switches to then? Yes, that's right ... your stored fat reserves.

So here are your options:

- Eat a diet high in refined carbohydrates, exercise intensely and for incredibly long periods until the supply is diminished, allowing you to then use fat reserves; or
- Consume the appropriate quantities of protein, fat and carbohydrates to allow your body to use stored body fat for fuel, not only from the minute you commence deliberate exercise, but with every movement you make throughout the day!

I'm sure the former approach would appeal only to masochists!

What does it take?

The following examples show some simple ways of making the 'energy balance equation' work in your favour. Remember, if you use your intellect you don't need willpower. These small changes, when combined, can make a huge difference!

- Drink a can of diet soda instead of one containing sugar – save 150 calories
- Skip with a rope for 7 minutes (or 7x1 min.) – burn 75 calories

Everyday for one month ... the result is improved fitness and a one kilogram fat loss.

- Eat a piece of fruit instead of a large glass of juice – save 100 calories
- Walk the dog for 30 minutes – burn 150 calories

Everyday for one month ... the result is improved fitness for you and your dog and a fat loss bonus for you of one kilogram.

- Cut out 2 slices of bread and butter/margarine – save 200 calories
- Walk 20 minutes to work and back – burn 200 calories.

The result is a 1.5 kilogram fat loss in one month and, of course, improved fitness (and maybe a less stressful day at work)!

A good example of an illogical approach to nutrition was evident when I was watching the introduction to a marathon on television. The commentator, also a well-known athlete, was explaining what the runners would experience during the lead up to the race. He said that they would all consume copious quantities of high-carbohydrate foods for a day or two prior to the race. On the morning of the event they would eat another refined carbohydrate meal and therefore would be feeling bloated and tired. However, they needed the energy supplied by these foods!

'Bloated and tired' – the commentator's words. Is that the way you would care to feel at the beginning of a race? If we listen to our bodies, and condition and fine-tune them with optimum nutrition, we would not need to feel this way in order to sustain energy. The commentator then went on to say that half-way through the run, most athletes would experience 'hitting the wall' – a common expression used by athletes to describe what it feels like when you run out of energy. If you have ever experienced this feeling, you would agree that it literally feels like you have run into a brick wall. How could this happen to such highly conditioned athletes? The answer is that as carbohydrate-loading bodies, they run out of immediate supply of carbohydrate fuel (glycogen). The human body is generally able to reserve around 800–1200 calories worth of glycogen. If the athletes rely on carbohydrates as their primary source of fuel, isn't it obvious that they would run out of fuel/energy in the middle of the race?

Many studies have been carried out on runners from primitive countries who still live primarily as hunter/gatherers. These guys seem to make excellent marathon and endurance athletes. Why? Because they appear to use stored fat reserves as their main source of fuel.

If a 70 kilogram male athlete has 10% body fat, this would indicate that he is carrying seven kilograms (10%) of his body weight in the form of stored fat. Remember that the value of 1 kilogram of fat is 7, 700 calories, therefore he would have enough reserved energy to sustain him through 53, 900 calories-worth of exercise. This is equivalent to approximately 90 hours of running, as opposed to the somewhat shorter duration of a marathon!

Now I hear you saying, 'But this is an athlete's diet you are describing ... and I'm not going to be using energy like an athlete does.' On the contrary, you obviously have far more available energy stored in the form of body fat than the elite athlete does.

The average 'healthy' woman may weigh 60 kilograms and be carrying around 25% of her weight in fat (15 kg).

15 kg x 7, 700 = 115, 500 calories.

So, theoretically, it is an ample quantity of calories to sustain 192.5 hours of running, or 385 hours of walking! If you were able to get through that amount of stored energy, you would be an extraordinary human being! *Think about it!* The less active we become, the fewer calories we need to consume, and this applies not only to total calorie consumption, but also to the type of foods those calories are composed of.

9
VITAMINS ... WHO NEEDS THEM?

Likc anything else in life, if you do not understand the reasons behind each choice that you make, even though you know 'you should' and 'it's good for you', sooner or later it becomes a chore, and then you quit!

I hope this chapter will simplify the subject of vitamins and minerals and put it in perspective. If you would like to have a more 'in-depth' look at vitamins, then the final chapter is for you.

Whether derived from food sources or supplementation, vitamins and minerals are essential to a healthy body.

Free health insurance, anyone?

It is popular opinion that if we eat a 'balanced diet', then taking vitamins or minerals in supplement form is a waste of time and money. If you were to analyse as many people's diets as I have, you would probably discover that 'balanced' is not the word to describe most of them. If we eat foods void of the necessary vitamins and minerals to help the metabolic process, then our metabolism will not be able to function effectively.

Vitamins help to convert the foods we eat into energy and living tissue, such as bones, muscles, blood, nerves and skin, and they enable the body to resist infection and protect our cells against disease. We are made up of trillions of tiny cells which are copied and replaced constantly. As old cells die off, we use the nutrients that we consume to rebuild and replenish supplies. Over a 24-month period, every cell in our body is replaced. These functions rely on the nutrition we choose to ingest.

The expression 'you are what you eat' could not be closer to the truth!

With the combination of modern-day, food-processing technology, food additives and preservatives, medications, hectic and stressful lifestyles (both physical and emotional) and environmental pollution, many essential nutrients are far from balanced in our diet.

Unless you live on a deserted island, with no contamination, no stress or pollution, perfect soil mineral content, grow your own food without sprays or additives and run a livestock farm, you may want to reconsider the meaning of the word balance.

The case for vitamin supplements

Vitamins and minerals, whether contained within our foods or in supplement form, are essential for normal growth and metabolism. We need them to remain healthy.

There seems to be a growing awareness of the relationship between vitamins and health benefits, beyond deficiency diseases. There is a vast contrast between remaining free of disease and achieving optimum health and wellbeing.

Well before signs of deficiency are obvious, immune system reactions have been significantly decreased.

The immune system may have a higher nutrient requirement than other organs and tissues of the body. For instance, before Vitamin A levels are low enough to create Vitamin A-related blindness in children their ability to fight infections has already been severely compromised.

For many years, physicians and scientists had been ignoring the effectiveness of vitamin and mineral preventative therapy, only to find, in the past decade, much of the research on supplements has confirmed their effectiveness.

The 2 major groups of vitamins are:

- fat-soluble vitamins – A, D, E, K and Beta-carotene
- water-soluble vitamins – B1, B2, B3, B5, B6, B12, C and Folate.

Who needs more than a little extra?

Recommended daily intake (RDI) amounts (by governments all around the world) are considered adequate to prevent medically-accepted nutritional deficiencies and related diseases, such as scurvy, beriberi, pellagra, rickets and anaemia. These RDIs do not address the increased need for nutrients required by:

- those who have chronic ailments
- those who are taking medication, including the contraceptive pill, antibiotics, anti-inflammatory drugs, anti-histamines, chemotherapy drugs, laxatives and some diuretics
- people who exercise regularly and require extra growth as a result of muscle breakdown, and more than normal recovery from the exercise itself
- smokers, or people who are subjected to stress, trauma and environmental pollutants
- elderly people who are often light eaters, or have difficulty preparing food
- alcohol drinkers – alcohol can inhibit absorption of some nutrients
- dieters on calorie restrictions, including many dancers and models
- teenagers who lead erratic lifestyles and tend to eat haphazardly.
- vegetarians (vegans) who may lack Vitamin b12 and iron
- children, who require optimum nutrition for growth and development
- those who consume commercially processed foods, or foods that have been sprayed or treated with chemical preparations.

You are probably thinking that this list covers just about the whole population. Well, you are right!

Vital nutrients may be lost from foods due to poor storage, exposure to air (oxygen can destroy some vitamins), over-cooking vegetables in water, thus creating a loss of water-soluble vitamins, and exposing foods to high temperatures for long periods of time.

Further research has proven that higher levels of certain vitamins are necessary for optimum health, and may also provide extra protection against cancer, heart disease and many other common ailments. In time, RDIs of vitamins may be broadened to include a much higher level to optimise their disease-preventing properties.

Some research that supports this involves Vitamin E, the RDI of which, in Australia to date, is only 10mg per day. In May 1993, the Harvard University School of Medicine published studies in the *New England Journal of Medicine* showing that Vitamin E supplements of over 100 mg per day reduced heart disease risk by over 40%.

A testimonial from Brigitte Duclos

Over the years I have consulted Donna for guidance and motivation to lose the odd kilo and keep myself on the healthy track. One memorable time in our training relationship was a fitness challenge from a national fitness magazine. I agreed to follow a diet and exercise regime designed by Donna for a period of 12 weeks. The magazine followed my progress for that period, after which I appeared on the cover – with great results, all thanks to Donna.

I had never considered myself fat but I was out of shape. Before starting Donna's plan I seriously doubted I had the willpower to stick with any plan but, despite the obstacles of a heavy workload and a fairly hectic lifestyle, Donna managed to structure a brilliant food plan and exercise format compatible with my schedule. The diet was a crucial part of this challenge – I had a relatively short time to lose body fat and increase muscle tone, but I needed maximum nourishment to keep me going.

Donna did for me what no one has been able to do before – she gave me the knowledge to work with my body and not against it – I've achieved results that I wouldn't have thought possible. She is a leader in her field.

This book is the next best thing to a clone of Donna in your handbag!

Brigitte Duclos is a television and radio personality.

Brigitte's statistics

Brigitte lost 10.19 kg of fat and gained 6.05 kg of muscle in 12 weeks.

Initial body fat – 33.43%   After 12 weeks – 18.24%

BMR after 12 weeks: + 196 calories a day

10
STOP THE CLOCK!

The ageing process ... can we slow it down?

Although we usually accept them as 'normal', ill health and/or weight gain do not have to be a natural part of the ageing process.

What are free radicals?

Every time you eat, oxygen is required to 'burn' this fuel, providing warmth and energy. Free radicals are a normal by-product of this process. They are also created when you expose yourself to sunlight, ozone, x-rays/radiation, tobacco smoke, fried foods/ processed fats and oils, emotional trauma, physical stress, exhaust fumes and exposure to the chemical additives in your food supply.

There is a war going on inside your body every minute of the day. Under normal circumstances, your defence troops (immune system and antioxidants) can handle the fight, however, if you become over-stressed or run-down, you'll become far more vulnerable to enemy attack. At high levels, free radicals can become quite a threat, contributing to many degenerative diseases.

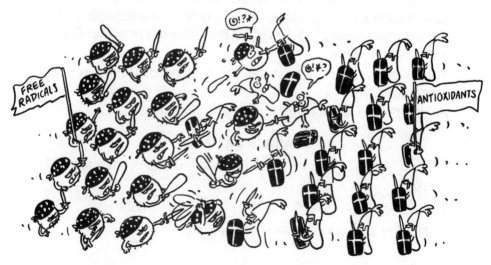

A distressing fact about free radicals is that they can harm you without the damage being visible!

The damage, rather than being overtly toxic, is eventually expressed as accelerated ageing or degenerative disease. Free radicals can be controlled within your body at low levels, however, if high levels are present, they are capable of destruction.

> We have all witnessed an apple turning brown after being exposed to oxygen. Unfortunately you can't immediately see the damage being done when *you* are becoming 'oxidised'!

If free radicals damage your DNA, an eventual consequence could be a higher risk of cancer. If free-radical damage occurs in your arteries supplying blood to the heart, it could eventually lead to a heart attack. Free radicals are now known to be involved in promoting cancer, heart disease, arthritis and, perhaps, as many as 80 diseases not caused by 'germs'.

> There are over 3,000 approved chemicals added to processed foods in America today, with an additional 10,000 chemical contaminants added unintentionally.

For this reason, it makes perfect sense to consume antioxidants in your food and/or as supplements to quench free radicals and minimise potential damage.

> Just as penicillin and antibiotics control the germs/bacteria that attack cells, antioxidants offer the same protection against free-radical attack.

The DNA in each cell can be 'hit' as many as 10,000 times a day by free radicals. Over a lifetime, unrepaired damage accumulates. This can cause unregulated growth of cells (tumours and other cell mutations).

Die old ... stay pretty!

Premature ageing is often a sign of diminishing 'healthy' cells in your body, promoted primarily by free-radical damage. It can cause proteins to link together (cross-linking) creating a 'stiffening' of the tissues. The result …ageing. Free radicals are capable of interfering with the absorption of nutrients and the elimination of waste from your cells, both of which will eventually kill them.

Antioxidants to the rescue!
Antioxidants are the brave soldiers forming your defence troops. They neutralise free radicals and prevent oxidation of fats, therefore preventing excessive damage. Research is still in its infancy, however, antioxidants have been shown to prevent or delay many disease processes, and to slow ageing.

Where do I find antioxidants?
Some of the most significant antioxidant vitamins are: Vitamins A, C, E and Beta-carotene. Minerals such as Selenium, Zinc and Manganese play important roles, as do various enzymes such as superoxide dismutase (SOD), co-enzyme Q10 and glutathione.

It is recommended that you consume a variety of antioxidants, not just a single one. As with all nutrients, they are most effective when a variety are present at one time. Many Australians do not get sufficient antioxidant nutrients from their diet. The demand dictated by your body is increasing due to lifestyle changes, as well as chemicals and pollutants in the environment and food supply.

If you're consuming an abundance of fresh vegetables, nuts and seeds, you may be covering your requirements. However, realistically, I think we could all confess to not consuming adequate vegetables on a consistent, daily basis.

How much is enough?
Well, everybody has varying requirements. If you were to eat a large salad at lunch time, consisting of four or five colorful vegetables, a large serving of steamed vegetables and a piece of fruit, you'd be well on your way! If you happen to be a smoker, under a lot of stress (physical or emotional), or worship the sun, you will almost certainly need more.

There is quite a difference between the recommended daily intake specified by government health authorities and those amounts recommended for optimum protective qualities as shown below:

Antioxidant vitamin	RDI	Protective quantity
Vitamin A	2, 500 IU	12, 500–25,000 IU
Vitamin C	40 mg	1000–18,000 mg
Vitamin E	15 IU	300–1600 IU
Beta Carotene	4.5 mg	15 mg

Good food sources and antioxidants

Beta-carotene – leafy greens (kale, mustard, collard), squash, capsicum, avocado, oranges, pawpaw and all fruit and vegetables with dark green, orange, red and yellow coloring.

Vitamin A – liver, cod liver oil, butter, cheese, yoghurt and milk.

Vitamin C – kiwifruit, papaya, brussel sprouts, strawberries, blackberries, raspberries, cauliflower, cabbage, grapefruit, capsicums, mandarins.

Vitamin E – unrefined vegetable oils, fresh nuts and seeds, wheat germ oil and wheat germ, sunflower seeds, almonds, hazelnuts, avocado, egg yolk, walnuts, fresh peanut butter, leafy greens (fresh spinach, kale), fish and shellfish, mangoes, whole grains.

Selenium – cashew nuts, halibut, meat, oysters, salmon, scallops, tuna, eggs and garlic.

Lycopene – tomatoes and tomato products, watermelon, red grapefruit and guava.

Lipoic acid – spinach, broccoli, brewer's yeast and muscle and organ meats.

Oligomeric proantho-cyanidins (OPC's) – grape skins, grape seeds.

You can live longer ... 5 easy-to-follow ways to make a difference!

1 Know what you are eating!

Choose to eat clean, real foods. Much of our food supply is contaminated. Between 1990 and 1995, the USA Environmental Protection Agency permitted 454 fertiliser companies to recycle and use in manufacturing, 271 million pounds of toxic waste, including lead and arsenic. Imagine eating food grown in that!

It is becoming more difficult to avoid toxic mess-ups such as these, but it is crucial to steer away from processed foods, trying to aim for organic, fresh fruit and vegetables wherever possible.

2 Consume plenty of the antioxidant nutrients

Whether in the form of fresh foods or supplementation, a balance of antioxidant nutrients is essential for preservation of your health and your youth.

3 Exercise!

How much is enough? As a rough guideline, the average person should aim to achieve a total of a least 5 hours exercise per week. Depending on different lifestyles and abilities, this may include walking, weight-training, tennis ... or a combination of various activities.

4 Maintain a strong immune system

This is your body's defence against pollutants and disease. You can do many things to enhance your own immune system. If your immune response becomes suppressed because it has worked so hard at protecting you from an unhealthy lifestyle and diet, it will not be capable of protecting you when you really need it. It only has a certain amount of 'man-power' available. If you force your body to use your defences haphazardly, and unnecessarily, you will have no troops left to fight 'real diseases' when they threaten you!

Here are some tips on how you can help:

- Eat a balanced, nutritious diet.
- Avoid excess stress.
- Protect your body from pollutants as much as possible.
- Make your rest, recovery and relaxation time a priority.
- Avoid the blasé approach to 'cure-all' drugs and antibiotics.
- Choose not to smoke.

5 'Let go' and enjoy yourself!

You only live once ... so make the most of it! So many of us spend our entire life preparing for the 'future', meanwhile we sacrifice our everyday present time in the process! Letting go and enjoying the present is a great stress release.

Both physical and emotional stress can play primary roles in the ageing process.

11
THE 'NITTY-GRITTY' ON FIBRE

Due to the evolution of food processing and convenient, prepackaged products, we seem to have overlooked one crucial component of our diet ... fibre!

We receive a great deal of information about the value of high-fibre foods, and there are masses of recipe books to teach us how to cook them. Unfortunately, to achieve an adequate fibre intake using much of this information means that we also consume copious quantities of processed carbohydrates. What foods do you immediately think of when I mention the word fibre?

Probably, wholegrain bread, cereals, muesli bars and rice would come to mind. How on earth are we supposed to consume the quantity of fibre recommended for optimum health, yet strive to keep our carbohydrate intake from becoming excessive? After all, they seem to be one and the same foods, don't they?

What are the best sources of fibre?
Soluble fibres like pectin and guar, form gels in water and prolong the transit time of material through the intestines allowing time for nutrients to be efficiently absorbed. The best sources of soluble fibre are fruits and vegetables, oat bran, psyllium husks and flaxseed. Insoluble fibres such as cellulose tend to reduce transit time. The best sources of insoluble fibre are wheat bran, rice bran, nuts, seeds and the skin of fruits and vegetables.

Is fibre really that important?
The main function of dietary fibre is to exercise the intestinal walls to retain their health and tone, therefore assisting regular elimination. Fibrous foods also help satisfy the appetite.

Fibre may play a role in the management of medical problems such as obesity, constipation, diarrhoea, haemorrhoids, diverticulosis, colon cancer, raised blood lipids (fats), cardiovascular disease and diabetes. Low-fibre foods can take up to five times longer to pass through the digestive system (15 –75 hours). This can create stagnation in the digestive tract and sluggish elimination of waste from the body.

The recommended daily intake of fibre for adults is 30–40 grams per day. In the average Western diet today, people are consuming less than 10 grams per day ... even with diets high in carbohydrate content! How can this be? Two words .... food processing!

If I asked you to think of some fibre-rich foods, the list of commonly consumed foods, below, might come to mind. However, if you look at the preferred food sources list you will see some foods that might surprise you in their fibre content.

Commonly consumed foods	Preferred food sources
1 cup noodles (cooked)	1 apple
1 cup rice (cooked)	$\frac{1}{2}$ cup brussel sprouts
1 slice multi-grain bread	1 carrot
30 grams cornflakes cereal	30 grams almonds
Muesli bar	$\frac{1}{2}$ cup raspberries
Calories: 710	Caloriess: 550
Carbohydrate: 144 gm	Carbohydrate: 35 gm
Fibre: 6.2 gm	Fibre: 22.1 gm

The aim of this comparison is not to have you literally substitute each item in the first list with the corresponding one in the second, but to make you aware that you can only have optimum nutrition if you have the knowledge. This comparison indicates that you don't have to consume high-carbohydrate foods to include adequate fibre in your daily diet. Many nuts, seeds, brans and husks are very low in carbohydrates and extremely high in fibre, not to mention numerous essential vitamins and minerals. For example:

Food source	Quantity	Carbohydrate grams	Fibre grams
Psyllium Seed Husks	2 tblsp (10 gm)	1	8
Linseeds	2 tblsp (25 gm)	1	6
Sesame Seeds	2.5 tblsp. (30 gm)	1	8
Pumpkin Seeds	2.5 tblsp. (30 gm)	5	3
Almonds	25-30 nuts (30 gm)	1	4.3
Wheat Germ	2 tblsp. (15 gm)	5	3
Wheat Bran	2 tblsp. (10 gm)	2	6.5

Before you screw up your nose at the idea of dining with your pet budgie, you will discover that many of the above foods can add flavour and texture in food preparation and baking, and don't necessarily have to be eaten by the handful.

Without you even noticing their existence, you will still reap the benefits of their superior nutritional qualities.

Reducing carbohydrates in our eating regime is often criticised by 'diet experts'. They will commonly argue that you will be eliminating essential nutrients and fibre. There are many unprocessed food sources that can be incorporated into a lower-carbohydrate diet, offering both high nutritional value and more than enough fibre.

Fresh vegetables, nuts and seeds supply fewer calories and carbohydrates than foods traditionally thought of as high-fibre, yet successfully supply more essential nutrients than the processed states of bread, rice and commercial cereals combined!

12
CHOLESTEROL

Dangerous fat in your blood ... or essential for well being?

The subject of cholesterol is surrounded by controversy. The common belief is that the lower our total cholesterol, the healthier we are! Think again.

What is cholesterol?

Cholesterol is a white or pale yellow, almost insoluble substance found in all animal tissues, blood, bile, and animal fats.

With all the publicity in recent years, most of us associate high cholesterol levels with disease, but how many of us know what it actually does? Very few people realise that cholesterol is an essential component of a healthy body. At present, it seems to be treated as a foreign, toxic substance causing disease. In fact, unexplained falling cholesterol levels are considered a grave sign, often being a marker for cancer.

Why do we need it?

The body needs cholesterol to maintain the health of all cell membranes and to control the flow of nutrients in and waste products out. Cholesterol assists in the absorption of fat-soluble Vitamins, A, D, E and K from our food, as well as giving our skin the ability to shed water. I could go on mentioning its varied functions, but I think you get the picture!

The average diet includes approximately two cups of refined carbohydrates per day, yet to eat a 'high-cholesterol' egg is bad for your health?

Without going into too much detail, there is a lot more to the cholesterol saga than the old cholesterol theory allows for. It was once thought (and still is by many), that if you eat a high fat diet you will have high cholesterol, yet if you eat a very low fat diet you won't. It sounds very simple, yet why are there so many exceptions to this rule? Going back to the out-dated food pyramid illustrated earlier, there is no discrimination between fats that are essential to health and those responsible for health decline. Is it really the amount of cholesterol-containing foods we eat that creates the problem, or is it how our body processes the cholesterol once it is in our system? Only 20% of our intake of cholesterol is supplied through our food. The remaining 80% is manufactured within the liver. We can use and replenish up to 2000mg of cholesterol per day.

Cholesterol is transported around the body in vehicles known as lipoproteins.

- *High-density lipoproteins* (HDLs)) are known as *'good'* cholesterol, because they return unused cholesterol to the liver, therefore removing it from our bloodstream and arteries.
- *Low-density lipoproteins* (LDLs) are known as *'bad'* cholesterol, because they carry cholesterol away from the liver, into the bloodstream where it is often found forming 'plaque' in our arteries. This eventually constricts the blood flow and puts us at risk of heart attack.

One very important factor overlooked in many theories, is that LDL is only left to form plaque in the arteries if it has been oxidised. Simply, this means that it becomes rancid. This happens as a result of inadequate antioxidant nutrients, too many processed fats and not enough essential fats. Its altered structure cannot be picked up and returned to the liver, influencing scavenger cells in the artery walls to take up the damaged LDL. Our immune system sends white blood cells to rid the arteries of damaged LDL deposits, creating a white, 'foamy'substance. If the amount of LDL exceeds our immune systems response, then plaque will begin to build on artery walls, obstructing blood flow.

What price are we paying by trying to be 'healthy'?

Deficiencies in many B vitamins, calcium and iron exist, particularly among women and children, due to reduced consumption of meat, eggs, cheese and other dairy products. We eat fewer of these foods today because of the international panic about consuming meats, fats and other cholesterol/fat containing foods. Heart associations and other medical authorities worldwide are ingraining this concern. These foods are considered taboo, yet what of all the people who have religiously adhered to the 'low-fat' way of life but continue to have the same old problems with their health and their weight?

Our increased intake of dietary fat is said to be the reason behind our increase in heart disease. Since 1964, our animal-fat intake has only increased by 6%, while the intake of vegetable fats has escalated by 160%. If fat has been the culprit over the last few decades, it must have been due to vegetable fat, not animal fat. Think about all those highly-processed, commercial vegetable oils on the supermarket shelves!

Blood triglycerides (fats) have been shown to increase on a low-fat diet by more than 32% due to an increase in carbohydrate consumption!

If we consume a diet higher in any form of calories than we can use (protein, carbohydrate or fats), the excess will be converted to triglycerides and be transported for storage. Many carbohydrate food sources are concentrated in calories (particularly sugar-laden foods), therefore the excess carbohydrate is unused and available for conversion to triglycerides.

The so called 'heart-healthy' butter replacements, such as margarine, should now be put on your most dangerous foods list (see trans-fatty acids in the chapter on further reading). These fats can considerably increase your risk of heart disease, along with numerous degenerative diseases.

Defying the traditional theory
The French consume a diet very high in fat (average of 44% of calories), yet they have one-third the heart disease of America. The French supermarkets, as with many other European countries, are not full of the latest fat-free wonder products; at least not to the

extent of the American or Australian shops. Instead, they tend to market high quality, fresh and unprocessed real foods.

The Eskimos have long been known for their high intake of fatty fish and blubber. Their fat consumption is estimated to be as high as 70% of their total calories, yet they have a very low incidence of heart disease or other health problems related to a high-fat diet. The fats they consume are fresh, natural and have not been altered or tampered with by man. This evidence should be enough to make us re-evaluate the current, popular belief about fat intake.

13
MYTHS AND MISCONCEPTIONS

This chapter is devoted to answering some of the most commonly asked questions regarding health, fitness, weight control and this program.

Q: 'I think I have a slow metabolic rate. Is this why I have so much difficulty controlling my weight?'

A: Perhaps you do have a slow metabolic rate, however, it is probably not for the reason you think! Many people seem to be under the impression that as we age, it is our unavoidable destiny to gain fat ...Wrong! Unless you have been diagnosed with a rare medical condition, the major causes of a lowered metabolic rate are inactivity and yo-yo dieting. These factors both create a reduction of lean tissue – the very thing that dictates the intensity of our inner furnace/metabolism.

Sorry to burst your bubble, but you are going to have to re-evaluate this one! As soon as you accept responsibility for your own health and wellbeing you will be empowered. As long as you blame someone or something else you will not be able to take control and create change. If your desire is to lose an excess of stored body fat and it's not happening, then you need to make changes in your current diet and become a little more active. It's that simple!

Q: 'If I train with weights in the gym, will my muscles get too big?'

A: It takes big weights to build big muscles. Even if, as a beginner, you were, to lift the heaviest weight you could physically handle, it would still not be heavy enough to create much increase in muscle size.

Muscle tone is a term that applies to the amount of tension in the muscle. If a muscle is not exercised it will deteriorate, becoming flaccid and loose. Sometimes women comment that their legs become big from weight training very quickly, so they prefer not to train them with weights. If you are carrying a large percentage of body fat and begin a weight training program, your muscles may appear larger. This is due to the fat over the surface of the muscle, as well as intramuscular fat. Thighs are the common area that women will retain most of their fat cells, therefore it is usually a problem area to 'tone-up'. Men, on the other hand, carry most of their fat on the abdomen. Instead of dialling that 1-800 number to order your 'butt and thigh sculptor', I think it would be more advantageous to first learn the basic anatomy of your body.

If you look at a steak which is marbled with fat, alongside a very lean eye-fillet, you will see the difference between lean muscle (the eye-fillet) and muscle that contains a high level of body fat (marbled). As you become leaner, you will notice that your muscles appear tighter and more compact (smaller). This is due to fat loss from within the muscle itself. This is why body composition, not just weight loss, is crucial in reshaping your body. If you are eating correctly and pursuing a higher level of daily fat-burning activity, your muscles will take on a more streamlined appearance.

Exercising your legs can trim down your tummy!

Your leg muscles are amongst the largest muscles in your body, therefore they make up a large percentage of your lean weight. When these muscles are exercised and well-developed, they will enhance your entire fat-burning furnace and help you lose everywhere!

Most women do not have the hormone levels required to build any significant size in muscle tissue. Men are capable of a higher level of muscular development due to higher testosterone levels. If you are a 'genetic freak' and do begin to grow larger muscles than desired, all you have to do is stop increasing the weights used and focus on lighter weights and higher repetition. In all of my years of training people, including many athletes, I have yet to meet the freak!

Q: 'If I stop exercising, will my muscles turn into fat?'
A: This question is based upon a very commonly held misconception and is a physical impossibility. Muscle is working tissue, which is attached to our skeleton to serve the purpose of moving our body around. Fat is inactive, stored energy, which has not yet been used by the body. They are completely different cells. It would be like a hair turning into an eyeball. It can't happen!

This misconception probably evolved from seeing athletes quit competitive training and gain weight. Simply, they stop stimulating the muscle to grow and develop, cease intense training, yet continue to consume the same quantity of food as when they were training. The result …loss of muscle/lean tissue and increased storage of unused energy … body fat! Muscle will develop to adapt to the amount of resistance you apply to it. It will grow to accommodate the weight that you lift. If the stimulation changes or disappears your muscles will mirror this.

Q: 'If I do more sit-ups, will this help me to 'spot reduce' the fat from my abdominal area?'
A: It is not possible to 'spot-reduce' body fat. It would be more effective to increase general activity, therefore burn more calories. Fat is reduced in a general pattern all over the body. To single out an area for reduction would be as impossible as trying to make your car use petrol from the left side of the tank! As discussed in the answer above, fat and muscle are two very different things. To work a particular muscle that lies beneath a layer of excess stored energy (fat) is not going to stimulate fat-burning in that area. The routine performance of resistance exercises for the entire body, will increase general muscle tissue, therefore creating a larger furnace for fat burning. Fat may appear never to budge from the areas containing more fat 'storage tanks'. These are just thicker fat layers than in other areas, therefore it seems to take a lot longer to reduce. It will happen if you stick at it …consistency is the key!

Q: 'Every woman in my family has solid, heavy legs. Does this mean that I am stuck with the genetic traits my family history dictates?'
A: Genetics and hormones influence the way in which our fat cells are distributed throughout the body. Some people may have more

storage cells on the thighs, others may have them around the waistline. It is true that if you gain body fat you will gather most of it around these predetermined areas, however, it is still up to you whether you fill these cells or not! If you remain lean and healthy, there is no reason for you to accumulate excess fat anywhere. There are many strong genetic influences in your body's chemistry, but the bottom line is that the individual lifestyle that you choose will determine your body composition, not your mother, sister or brother!

Q: 'Are some carbohydrate foods better than others? If so, what are the differences?'

A: How many people do you know who *don't* want value for money? Getting our money's worth is very important to us and exactly the same attitude should apply to getting our 'calories worth' of nutrition. We should want 'value for calories'. For example, the average carbohydrate content of a chocolate bar is approximately 50 grams, with calories in excess of 300 and very little nutritional value or fibre. I have no doubt that you would still be hungry an hour after consuming this snack. In comparison, to consume the same quantity of calories and carbohydrate in a vegetable, you would need to pile about 1 kilogram of it onto your plate. The value of vitamins, minerals and nutrients derived from vegetables is astounding, not to mention the volume and fibre (over 60 grams of fibre). I am not suggesting that you eat 1 kilogram of broccoli as your next snack, however, I hope this extreme example, illustrates the importance of getting value for calories.

The general rule in choosing the best carbohydrate foods is to choose only 'real food'. How do you know if it's real? Ask yourself a simple question. 'Did it grow that way, or was it manmade?'

You cannot go out into a field and pick a loaf of bread, pasta or cereal. You can pick wheat, but there is no way your system can digest it until it has been highly processed, removing most of the nutritional value and fibre along the way. I cannot say this often enough – the easy guideline is to stick with real foods, such as fibrous vegetables, nuts, seeds and low-carbohydrate, high-fibre fruits.

Q: 'I have cellulite all over the back of my thighs. I have tried all the creams, pills and diets, yet none of them seems to help. Is it possible to get rid of the dimpled appearance?'
A: It is absolutely possible to rid your body of the dimpled fat commonly known as cellulite. Cellulite is fat … period! Many product manufacturers would like you to believe that it is a dreaded disease, caused by 'toxic build-up' or 'poor circulation'. Of course, their product is 'just the thing' to cure it!

The cellulite myth … banished now and forever!

A short time prior to the release of this book I was involved in a research project with HSV 7, a television station in Melbourne, testing a popular 'cellulite treatment' pill. I was so disturbed by a story on Channel 7 which seemed to be promoting these pills as an instant miracle-cure, that I wrote a letter to the producer of the program offering some factual information that would show the pills to be a 'gimmick' superbly marketed by manufacturers and advertisers who are only too aware of how fragile and vulnerable females are when it comes to body image.

The producers accepted the challenge and we ran a trial involving three women who took the pills daily for eight weeks. We assessed their body composition with an ultrasound machine to observe any changes in body fat. There was no evidence that the cellulite pill created any fat loss. I initiated a comparative study on a another woman using nutrition and light exercise to achieve a loss of cellulite. Within eight weeks, our subject had lost 5 kilograms of fat and gained 1 kilogram of lean weight, boasting a significant reduction in 'cellulite' from her upper thighs! (See 'Helen's testimonial', Chapter 15.)

This dimpled appearance, usually on the upper thighs and bottom, is due to a thicker area of body fat than elsewhere. In other words, the thicker our fat beneath the skin becomes the heavier it is, the more it bulges outwards against our skin, showing itself as dimpled pockets. Excess body fat accumulates in these areas because more fat cells (storage tanks for excess fat) are located there. This process is both preventable and reversible. To banish 'cellulite', you need to change your body composition. This means an increase in lean tissue (muscle) and a decrease in stored fat. Let's say it all together now … 'The only way to achieve this is to make changes to your current diet and activity regime!'

Q: 'Why do most women have cellulite on their thighs but not on their tummies where they often have a lot of body fat, and why is it so much easier to lose tummy fat?'

A: Fat cells on the thighs and bottom are more abundant in women than in men due to our hormones. The very hormones that make our bodies capable of child-bearing also dictate the fat storage areas in our bodies. Fat stored between the waist and the knees is more resilient to diet and exercise because it is accumulated there as a protective mechanism in anticipation of pregnancy and lactation. Studies have shown that fat is mobilised from these areas during pregnancy and lactation, and stubbornly stays put the rest of the time! When lack of muscle tone is present in the thigh area, the dimpled appearance of this fat will be more pronounced. Female hormones also make our skin finer and thinner than men's therefore thickened areas of fat cells are more apparent beneath the skin.

As for the lack of dimples in the abdominal area– this fat is not stored for use during child-bearing and is largely visceral fat (fat within the abdominal cavity and surrounding organs) as opposed to the subcutaneous fat on the limbs (directly beneath the skin). It is, however, quite possible for abdominal fat to show a dimpled appearance, but not as likely as on the thigh area. Visceral fat (apple shape) is more dangerous to our health than subcutaneous fat (pear shape).

Q: 'I have recently made changes in my diet, reducing a lot of refined and processed foods. Why am I feeling so fatigued? Do I need more carbohydrates to give me an energy boost?'

A: Your body may go through an adjustment period during the initial changes to your usual food intake. Firstly, you must be aware that you may have cut your calorie intake too far. If you were originally eating a high-carbohydrate diet and have now cut back on these foods, you must ensure that you replace these calories with the other better food sources. Your digestive tract will be required to manufacture different quantities of enzymes to digest the new foods you are eating. This process takes a little time to adapt, however, within a few weeks you should experience a higher energy level than ever before. The answer to this question also depends on the degree of change you have adopted. If you feel the change is too extreme to comfortably handle, you may want to reassess your goals and structure a gradual change, in weekly phases. You should also ensure that you are consuming enough calories to satisfy your nutritional needs. When we become more selective with our food choices, it is very easy to unintentionally cut total calories too far.

Q: 'Does too much protein harm the kidneys?'
A: Too much of anything is not going to create a balance in your diet, however, the answer is no, not if your kidneys are normal, healthy and free from disease to begin with. Do not assume that I am recommending an eating plan that is too high in protein. It may be higher than you are accustomed to, but if it were too high it would be more than your body can use. The quantity I recommend is based on the amount of lean mass you carry, therefore is certainly not too much. There are no findings of ill effects on the kidneys due to excess protein, assuming that the kidneys are functioning normally.

Q: 'I've been feeling dizzy and light-headed on this eating plan. Why?'
A: One possible cause for this feeling can be dehydration. Eating fewer carbohydrates than usual will stimulate the kidneys to release retained fluids. The solution to this is to ensure you drink plenty of fluids to replenish hydration. Most people do not consume enough water on any eating plan, but the effects are more noticeable on a lower-carbohydrate diet. You should never wait until you feel thirsty to drink, as this is usually a sign that you are already dehydrated.

Another reason for this light-headedness could be a reduction in total calories. Perhaps you have rearranged your food not realising that you have restricted your calories to a much lower level than your body is accustomed to. The feeling of dizziness could also be related to low blood-sugar levels, which can be a symptom of lowered calorie intake.

Q: 'I have been following your 'real food' plan for a few months now and I seem to have reached a plateau. Why, and what can I do to change this?'

A: Assuming that you have already achieved results to a certain point, I would suggest that your body has now adapted to your current regime of diet and exercise. Your body will always 'mirror' what you do. If you wish to create further changes, you may have to make adjustments. For example, you could slightly increase your daily activity. This may be enough to get the ball rolling again. Just remember – if you continue to put in the same amount of effort, you will continue to receive the same results! And, don't forget that changes to your body composition are not necessarily indicated accurately on the bathroom scales. You may gain muscle and lose fat, yet remain the same weight on the scales. For this reason, I suggest monitoring your progress in other ways. For example, with a body-composition test (callipers or ultra-sound, body-fat analysis), with a tape-measure or simply by the fit of your clothing. If you do not have access to a body-composition test facility on a regular basis (gymnasium, sports physician, etc), I recommend that you measure yourself with a tape every 4–6 weeks (circumference of waist, hips, thighs, upper arms).

If you feel you are definitely not changing, then keep an eye on your total calories. You may be eating more than you are burning off in activity. Or it may be that your carbohydrate intake is still too high to allow your body to use stored fat for energy. Perhaps it is a combination of the two. You certainly wouldn't be alone – this is a common error in judgement. It would be worthwhile to write down, as accurately as possible, what you are eating each day in order to calculate any error in your estimations of food intake. If you have developed the pattern of repeatedly restricting calories time and time again, on various diet plans, your body becomes very 'energy efficient'. In other words, after receiving that signal that you are starving to death in the middle of a desert, your body will do anything it can to preserve your life! It may take time and patience to re-educate your body. You will achieve this by persisting in following a sensible eating regime, eating the correct nutrients in the sufficient quantities and staying active.

Many of us over-estimate our activity and under-estimate our food intake. Studies have shown that when people who claimed that they were sticking to a particular food plan but not losing weight, were closely monitored to ensure they were eating exactly what they said they were eating, they did lose weight!

A testimonial from Rochelle Jackson

My testimonial about working out and eating following Donna's plan is simple – I say it works! In a mere 14 weeks I have lost six kg and a significant amount of fat. I have noticed a real change in the shape of my body and have gone from a substantial, curvaceous, size 14 to a svelte size 12 and I feel fantastic!

Although I have always exercised – daily aerobics classes, fun-runs, walking, pumping iron – I managed to keep fit, but could never alter my bodyshape or slim down, no matter how I sweated! I really wanted to lose about eight kg.

Starting on Donna's regime made me feel as if I had rediscovered the wheel! And my enthusiasm comes from success. Since starting with Donna I have totally changed my eating habits. My diet is now protein-based rather than carbohydrate – I eat nuts and protein bars and I drink protein shakes, and I'm eating meat for the first time in 15 years and thoroughly enjoying it.

My body has actually changed from being very pear-shaped and 'hippy' to a more hour-glass shape with significant weight-loss around my bottom, hips and waist. At the risk of sounding like a television commercial, I must say that my friends have noticed the difference and I feel great – more energy, and more confidence knowing that I am at last able to control what I put in my mouth and how I look. I've put the 'large gal' I once was behind me!

I have been so inspired by my new lifestyle that, at 34 years old, I'm considering competing in a bodyshaping contest – all thanks to Donna.

If the book is full of Donna's knowledge, ideas and enthusiasm then it can't help but be a great success.

Rochelle Jackson is a producer with the current affairs program Today Tonight *on television station, HSV 7*

14
OLD HABITS DIE HARD!

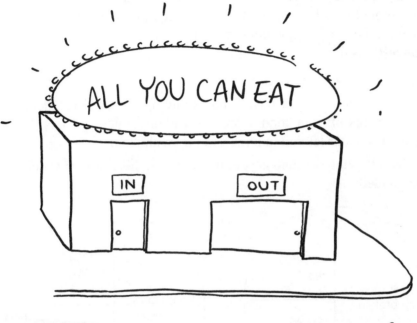

Planning your new pattern

With the information we have looked at so far, I think you are now ready to construct your own menu format, using this chapter as your guide.

Unlike almost every 'diet book' author, I have decided not to create a regimented menu plan that you must adhere to. Instead, I have supplied you with a sample menu planner if you feel that you require this type of structure, or you can use the knowledge you have gained, together with my own recipes, which follow. In my experience, regimented plans become impossible for most people to continue. The absolute principle of this book is to allow you the freedom to continue your busy career, and/or personal life, without becoming a frustrated social outcast with anti-social diet regimes. This knowledge should be incorporated into your lifestyle forever … not just for a three- or four-week 'quick-fix'.

Everybody has individual requirements, in calories, nutrition and food preferences. If you are wondering what to have for breakfast, you should now be able to check the following food listings and menu sample to assist your choice, or simply turn to the breakfast suggestions in the recipe section. It is designed to be easy.

So … What should I eat?

Now that you have a basic understanding of the three main components of your food – protein, carbohydrates and fats – I guess I'd better let you in on what to do with them!

If the following diagram is your dinner plate, this is how it should be divided:

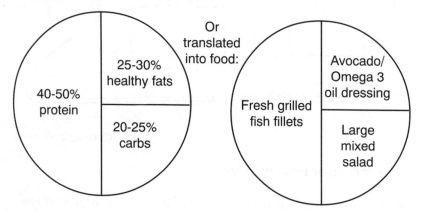

Protein

An easy calculation method is shown on the diagram above. Fill half of your dinner plate with protein foods. They consist of beef, poultry, fish and all seafood, lamb, pork, veal, organ meats, eggs, cheese, natural yoghurt (limited, due to some carbohydrate content) and protein powders (no added sugars). Be aware that some of your 'fat allowance' is contained within some protein foods.

Meats

Lean cuts of beef, lamb, pork or veal, including steaks, roasts, fillets, trim cuts or lean mince.

Ham, bacon and other processed or cured meats are alright occasionally, however, there are more nutritious alternatives in fresh produce.

Poultry and eggs

Chicken, turkey and other forms of poultry are excellent sources of protein. Be aware that the darker meats (leg, wing, etc.) and the skin are quite high in fat and calories, compared with the white meat of the breast.

Whole eggs are filled with a nutritious source of protein. If you are trying to reduce body fat, I would suggest you moderate your calories by excluding some of the yolks. If you were to make an omelette, for example, use one whole egg and four egg whites. The whites are rich in protein, yet only 15 calories each!

Fish

Fresh or tinned, fish is a great source of protein, as well as essential fats and oils. Salmon, tuna, prawns, oysters, lobster and all crustaceans are good choices. Beware of added carbohydrates in some commercial tinned fish products ... read the labels to be sure!

Dairy products

This category includes cheeses, cottage cheese, cream cheese, yoghurt, milk, cream and whey-protein powders. When selecting cheeses, be aware that some low-fat varieties do have carbohydrates added for texture. Milk should be limited due to the fact that it contains lactose, a natural milk sugar. Unsweetened or artificially sweetened yoghurt can be eaten in moderation, although, as with milk, it does contain lactose. Whey protein-concentrate powder can be purchased from any health food shop. It can make a convenient, healthy 'thick-shake' and contributes to many of the recipes in this book.

Carbohydrates

Carbohydrates, particularly nutrient-deficient, refined carbohydrates, are the least necessary component in a healthy diet and are over-consumed in most diets. If you are having trouble controlling your body-fat levels, I suggest that you try reducing all carbohydrates to around 25% of your total calories. If you are presently consuming 60% or more of your calories in the form of carbohydrates, you will have to increase other calorie sources significantly before you make this reduction. Keeping your carbohydrate percentage below 25% everyday will allow the fat-burning process to begin. This is quite a simple task if you keep the 'dinner plate' diagram in mind.

The entire purpose of this regime is to allow your body to burn the stored body fat that you have accumulated, for the purpose it was stored there in the first place – energy! At the same time, by choosing only the highest quality carbohydrate foods from the list provided, you will ensure more than adequate quantities of all nutrients and fibre required for optimum health.

Consume more ...
Low-carbohydrate/high-fibre, fresh vegetables
Asparagus, green beans, artichokes, broccoli, brussel sprouts, cabbage, capsicum, carrots, cauliflower, celery, cucumber, lettuce, mushrooms, onion, snow peas, spinach, silverbeet, spring onion, squash, zucchini.

Low-carbohydrate/high-fibre fresh fruits
Apples, apricots, avocadoes, tomatoes, strawberries, raspberries, cantaloupe, watermelon, grapefruit, passionfruit, peaches, pineapple.

Consume less ...
High-starch fruit and vegetables
Bananas, grapes, cherries, potatoes, peas, corn, sweet potato/yams.
Tinned, processed or dried fruit and vegetables.

Limit ...
Bread, rice, lentils, condiments and dressings containing sugars, milk, alcohol ... and even too many 'legal' carbohydrates!

Avoid ...
Foods that contain 'empty' calories, dried fruits, fruit or vegetable juice, flour and flour based products, pastry, biscuits, cakes, chips, sugar, fructose, honey, sugary drinks (including alcohol mixers), pasta, highly processed foods containing thickeners and sugars,

processed fats and oils (including those used in commercial cooking oils, muffins, biscuits, cakes, oil-roasted nuts etc), jams, donuts confectionery, chocolate, icecream and frozen yoghurt, potato crisps, pretzels and popcorn. These foods contain empty calories, processed fats or sugar, and, in most cases, all three! This is by no means a definitive list, but you get the general idea – repeat after me, 'Real food only!'

Fats

Fats should make up around 20–30% of your total calorie intake. You will discover that once you are consuming the right foods, this will regulate itself. Sure, you can add butter to your diet without guilt but what are you going to do with it? You won't be spreading it on your bread because you won't be eating bread! I think you will find that the fat percentage of your food will be adjusted automatically just by your consumption of protein foods, such as eggs, cheese, lean meat and nuts, with the addition of essential fatty acids from seeds, fish, oils or supplements. At least 12–15% of your total calories must be made up of essential fatty acids. This equates to approximately half of your daily fat consumption.

The 'fat-phobia'

There is a simple explanation for the increasing fear of eating fat. Low-fat food manufacturers spend exhorbitant amounts of money promoting their products and so must necessarily try to convince us that all fat is bad, bad, bad!

We must realise that low-fat foods are not necessarily healthy and nutrient dense. Before making a decision on the amount of fat you consume you should know that not every morsel of fat that you eat goes directly to your fat cells. The relationship between stored body fat, or unused energy, and fat contained in our foods is not as close-knit as we once thought. Because the caloric value of fat is greater than protein or carbohydrates, quite often those people eating a high-fat diet are also consuming more calories than they need. If you cut fat from your diet, then theoretically you will lose weight due to a cut in calories. By reducing your fat intake by 30 grams you should save yourself 270 calories. Unfortunately, there is a lot more to this premise. Firstly, most manufacturers of low-fat foods will add sugars and thickeners (carbohydrates) to their products to replace the taste and texture removed with the natural fats. This tends to increase the calories to the original amount, if not higher.

Fat makes us feel full and satisfied, therefore, we usually consume more low-fat foods to make up for this.

A person who consumes 2000 calories per day with 30 grams of fat will not lose weight faster than one who consumes 2000 calories with 60 grams of fat. 2000 calories taken in are 2000 calories to be burned!

Success lies in the ability to distinguish between the value of 'good' fats and oils, essential to health, and 'bad' fats which are detrimental.

Friendly fats and oils

All oils must be unrefined – olive oil, sesame oil, almond oil, walnut oil, macadamia oil, almonds, brazil nuts, pecans, hazelnuts, walnuts, pumpkin seeds, sesame seeds, sunflower seeds, macadamia nuts, pistachio nuts, all raw nuts and seeds, avocado, olives, fresh cream (unsweetened), butter, lecithin, and naturally occurring fats in meats, eggs, fish and dairy products.

From the categories listed, you will be able to formulate a flexible and convenient eating regime to suit your lifestyle and accommodate your individual likes and dislikes. Your appetite should regulate the quantities of food required once your body is nutritionally satisfied.

Water ... you can't drink too much of it!

Digestion, metabolism, temperature regulation, respiration, nutrient transportation, and elimination processes, all depend on the presence of water!

Only oxygen is more essential than water in sustaining your life. When the body over-heats, you have two-million sweat glands which excrete fluids that are 99% water. The evaporation of this perspiration helps to regulate your body temperature.

To function at an optimum level and to relieve stress on organs, the average adult requires approximately three litres of water to replenish supplies each day under normal circumstances. How much are you drinking?

Our water requirement is increased by strenuous exercise, warm climate or excessive salt intake. When there is a change in your food intake, particularly when reducing carbohydrate intake, your body will tend not to retain the fluids it used to. Reducing carbohydrates (and therefore insulin levels) causes a loss of retained fluid. Calorie reductions in general will also cause lower amounts of fluid because we derive much of our water from food. For this reason, you may have to increase your fluid intake by as much as 50%. I have said this before but it is worth repeating ... Do not wait until you feel the sensation of thirst to drink, because by this time, you are probably already dehydrated. Get into the habit of drinking plenty of fluids. If you consume any caffeine-based beverages, such as Diet Coke, coffee and tea, your requirement for fluids will increase, as they have a diuretic effect.

Sometimes, when you think you are hungry you are actually thirsty.

I can just picture some of you, as you read this statement, screwing up your faces knowing that – boy – you can sure tell the difference! It is, however, quite common for us to confuse the two.

Have you ever experienced a desire for something to eat, but you really can't decide what, and then you settle on a piece of fruit? It is likely that it is the high water content of the fruit that is appealing to your thirst.

You may want to start paying closer attention to the signals your body is sending to you. The next time you feel empty, ask yourself if you could possibly eat a meal, perhaps a steak or a chicken breast. If the answer is no, then have a large glass of water and within 30 minutes your desire will probably have diminished. Of course, if it is still there, then satisfy your hunger with a meal.

There is a vital connection between drinking water and fat loss. Why?

Water is required to assist the process of fat burning and elimination.

When you drink less than is required, the body feels threatened. In self-protection, it will retain fluid and be less efficient at fat burning.

By drinking water and correcting fluid retention, more fat is used as fuel because the liver is free to metabolise fat at top speed.

The kidneys cannot function well without enough water. When they do not work to capacity, some of their load is 'dumped' on the liver, forcing it to metabolise less fat.

Water helps wash out by-products of metabolism, prevents accumulation of body toxins, aids in the control of body temperature and electrolyte balance, and prevents constipation.

Tea, coffee and other beverages

Beverages such as tea and coffee can be consumed in moderation with just a splash of milk if desired and artificial sweeteners only. Some people tend to be more sensitive to caffeine than others and their blood-sugar levels may be more dramatically effected. If you feel this may apply to you, yet you love your cup of coffee, then switch to a decaffeinated product.

Fruit juices should be avoided at all times. Even if they have no added sugar, they are composed of fruit, minus the fibre. The average 250 mL glass of fresh orange juice contains approximately 25 grams of carbohydrate. Much of the vitamin and mineral content is destroyed within a very short time of being extracted from the fruit, leaving you with a glass of insulin-stimulating sugar! It would be far more beneficial to your health to consume the whole fruit in its natural state.

Diet sodas are perfectly legal as they contain no sugar. They must contain only artificial sweeteners, such as Nutrasweet, and no other form of carbohydrate. Some 'diet' beverages are labelled 'no added sugar', however contain, for instance, fruit juices.

Alcohol can be consumed in moderation. By moderation, I mean a glass of dry white or red wine with your meal. Any spirits consumed must also be in moderation and never with sweet mixers. You can choose 'on the rocks' or a diet mixer, such as diet cola or diet tonic, or soda water. All alcohol consumption must be factored into your daily calorie intake.

For the 'sweet-tooth'
Some 'legal' and 'not-so-legal' treats …

Icecream: There are very few commercially available, low-carbohydrate icecreams. Do not be seduced by low-fat products that remain high in sugars. Even sugar-free icecream should be seen as a treat and consumed accordingly.

Frozen yoghurts are usually high in sugar, even if they are low in fat. 'Vitari' has no added sugar, however, it is made from fruits, which are 100% refined carbohydrates, completely devoid of the fibre and essential nutrients normally found in fresh fruits.

Cream may be eaten occasionally. If it has been whipped commercially or in a restaurant, it will almost certainly contain sugar. You may whip fresh cream yourself and add artificial sweetener (Equal or Splenda). Remember, if you are trying to reduce body fat, you must take the very high calorie content of the cream into consideration.

Diet jelly is an excellent dessert or sweet indulgence. It is not exactly what I call real food, however, it is a harmless treat when you have a bit of a 'sweet tooth'. It is available in many flavours and is very low in both carbohydrates and calories.

Protein powder: Always choose a brand with no added sugars. This is a quick, easy and versatile source of protein. I have used it in many of my recipes to add flavour and texture, as well as to balance the nutritional proportions.

Sweeteners: Equal or Nutrasweet are the better alternatives. They are made from two amino acids (components of protein) and they do not have the significant after-taste associated with the various chemical-sweetening substances. For cooking you must choose a sweetener designed for cooking, such as Splenda. Equal is destroyed by the heat of cooking, losing all of its sweetness. Do not use sugar, honey, jam or any other high-carbohydrate-based sweeteners. Be aware that there are many forms of sugar, including fructose, maltose, dextrose, sucrose. Remember that even if a food label claims to be sugar-free, the product may still contain carbohydrates from other sources!

Sauces and dressings: Once again, read those labels and be aware of added sugars, starches and processed fats in salad dressings and condiments. Even better, make your own, then you can be assured that the best ingredients are used. Balsamic vinegar, lemon juice and/or fresh, unrefined oils can make excellent salad dressing.

15
WHY? HOW? WHAT? AND WHERE?

Why can't I eat starchy foods ... just fewer of them?

Obviously, if you choose a selection of the lowest carbohydrate, 'real' foods available, you will be able to consume a greater volume of food for the same carbohydrate value. If you decided to choose a banana at 40 grams of carbohydrate, you must realise that this may be almost half of your daily allowance, therefore you may have to go without many other foods throughout the day. Not only does this fail to satisfy your hunger, but it is also nutritionally unbalanced. On the other hand, you could eat a whole punnet of vitamin-rich strawberries for a mere 6–8 grams of carbohydrate.

It is all about balance. I recommend that most people consume no more than two pieces of fruit per day, although it depends on what percentage of their total calories this becomes. To explain this concept, if you ate only one apple in a day, but it was the only thing you ate all day, you would have eaten 100% carbohydrates for that day. Your goal is 25% carbohydrates. If you ate 2000 calories in a day, then the 100 calories of an apple would only equate to 5% ... got it?

How to make 'habit changes' simple

The recipes in this book are designed for you to simply construct tasty and satisfying meals in the correct proportions. Quite often, when making changes in our food plan, we lose our creativity in preparation by being cautious. You will soon discover a wide variety of recipes, which can be created from 'legal' foods. Instead of denying yourself the 'treats' you are accustomed to, just find a legal substitute. In my experience, I have not come across a recipe challenge yet that I could not meet with an alternative or substitute, tasting just as good, if not better!

Keeping a record of the foods you eat, as well as the fluids you consume on a daily basis will give you a much more accurate perspective. It is amazing what you learn about your eating patterns when they are actually written down in front of you. You will soon see a pattern relating to results, or lack of them!

I am not suggesting that you weigh every morsel of food you prepare, however, if you weigh your foods for a week or two, you soon develop an eye for estimating quantities.

What about vegetarians?

If you happen to be a vegan, then I'm afraid you will find it very difficult to find sufficient sources of quality protein to compose 50% of your calories. If this is the case and you don't wish to make any changes in this area, then I suggest you follow as much of the 'healthy lifestyle' approach recommended in this book as possible. You can still be aware of friendly fats and oils, antioxidants and nutrient balance, as well as trying to combine as much 'real food' as possible to create a balanced intake. Many vegetarians do consume dairy products and/or eggs. This would allow very easy adaptation to my menu planner.

Where do my family and children fit in? Can they follow the same regime?

Absolutely! For a start, I don't think it would be detrimental to anyone's health, regardless of age, to cut refined and processed foods from their diet. Elimination of sugars and trans-fatty acids from the diet is certainly not the cause of ill health in anyone I know of! The reason this diet is so easy to follow is the 'real food principle'. Yes, that's right, that fresh stuff you can go and buy at the market! As long as you don't restrict your children's calories by cutting out any nutritional foods, then it can only benefit them to eat a balanced diet of unprocessed foods. If you use your creativity in the kitchen, with the assistance of my recipes, your cooking may even gain a few more fans!

Before starting

If you have any health concerns before beginning this plan, then please be sure to consult your physician and let him or her know your intentions. If you are taking any medication, your doctor may want to test you on a regular basis to ensure the doses are still appropriate. If you are not on medication, it is still advisable to have a medical check up before commencing any lifestyle and dietary changes … even if it is only to supply you with a baseline. This can be used over time to show an improvement in your general state of health, or simply as a preventative measure.

What changes can I expect?

Your initial goals and your starting point will obviously influence the degree of change. You can expect your body's response to mirror the changes you adopt. In other words, the more changes you make, the more results will be evident. If you reach a plateau at any time, yet you feel you are still adhering to your regime quite well, you may only require the slightest alteration – perhaps an extra 15-minute walk a day, to start the ball rolling again. It need not necessarily be any more difficult than your current routine, just different! After a few weeks of making conscious changes, your new routine will become just as simple as the old one!

If you follow this regime correctly, some of the changes you will observe include:

- an improvement in skin texture due to the addition of essential fats, protein and other vital nutrients
- an increase in energy levels
- changes in body composition – more tone, more lean tissue, less body fat (therefore less dimpling of the skin)
- improvement in abnormal blood sugar, blood pressure and many other ailments
- a diminishing of cravings
- an improvement in the strength of fingernails and hair
- a large boost to self-esteem!

A testimonial from Helen Alfa

When I met Donna in November 1998, I hadn't really exercised for more than two years. In the past I have worked in the fitness industry, so I am no stranger to diet and exercise programs and the bewildering amount of conflicting information available.

I was quite excited and motivated to recommence regular training, although, at the same time, I was aware of how quickly that enthusiasm can disappear if you don't get results.

I am 32 years old and my career had been my top priority for some time. As a result I had let my health and fitness go a little. I was still in what I would consider a normal weight range but I wasn't as fit and toned as I would like. In the past dieting consisted of limiting calories with all the focus on reducing dietary fats to almost zero!

Then along came Donna with her radically different ideas about achieving maximum nutrition from 'real' food instead of poor nutrition from 'empty' food that not only had very little goodness, but also stopped you from successfully losing weight! Donna had me eating more protein, essential fats and much larger servings than any diet that I had ever been on allowed. Imagine, a diet where I didn't have to go hungry!

Almost immediately I noticed that my usually dry skin felt softer. By the third week the most prominent difference was the changing shape of my bottom and the definition in my abdominal area. Other diets would cause weight-loss in my face and upper body, but my proportions never seemed to alter. Donna explained that this was the difference between losing 'fat' and losing weight.

Just prior to Christmas 1998, I opened my restaurant, Jackie O, in Melbourne. Opening night was a very important event for me so it was a wonderful experience to feel so good and so confident. I wore a fitted dress with none of my former self-consciousness and the compliments were the icing on the cake (Donna's fabulous cheesecake of course!).

After only six weeks, the change in my shape was very obvious. My arms were defined and lean, tummy flat, bottom toned and in proportion, and thighs I finally felt proud of. No more wobbly bits!

I must admit that I did focus and make a concentrated effort and I believe that, as with most things, the results are dependent on how much you are willing to put in. However I have never found a more effective, more healthy method of achieving weight loss. Within eight weeks I lost 5 kg of fat and gained 1 kg of muscle, reducing my body fat from 26% to 17%.

Today, I feel that I have more control over my body – its weight, its shape and its health.

Helen Alfa is a restaurant proprietor.

Helen's statistics

Body-fat measurements

	11 Nov '98	*16 Dec '98*	*11 Jan '99*
Tricep	13 mm	10 mm	10 mm
Ab	20 mm	14 mm	10 mm
Thigh	14 mm	11 mm	10 mm
Weight	58 kg	56 kg	54 kg
Fat	25.87%	19.84%	17%

Total weight loss on scales: 4 kg

Total fat loss: 5 kg

Total lean gain: 1 kg

Total overall body fat lost (thickness of fat under skin): 17 mm.

16
YOUR BASIC MENU PLANNER

The following menu example shows a completely balanced structure covering all the necessary daily nutrients in correct proportions.

BREAKFAST

Protein milkshake: 150 mL skim milk

100 mL cold water

50 grams whey protein concentrate powder (WPC)

50 grams raspberries (fresh or frozen)

Equal sweetener to taste (optional)

Blend all ingredients to create a healthy breakfast shake.

MORNING SNACK

25 grams of raw almonds

LUNCH

Tuna salad: unlimited mixed salad greens

1 large ripe tomato, diced

red capsicum, diced

green capsicum, diced

150 grams tuna (water packed, drained)

100 grams light cottage cheese

25 grams sesame seeds

Combine all ingredients and dress with balsamic vinegar &/or fresh lemon juice.

AFTERNOON SNACK
1 cup fresh strawberries
sugarfree jelly (optional)

DINNER
Steak and vegetables
 250 grams lean, eye-fillet steak
1.5 cups of mixed vegetables, e.g. cauliflower, carrots, brussel sprouts

EVENING
20 grams hazelnuts
100 grams yoghurt (no added sugar)
30 grams whey protein concentrate (WPC)

*Mix WPC powder into the yoghurt to create a creamy dess*ert.

This sample menu has a nutritional breakdown of 50% protein, 20% carbohydrates and 30% 'healthy' fats.

The nutritional analysis for this menu plan is illustrated in the following graph. The graph indicates that the menu is designed to cover every nutrient mentioned, to at least 100% of the National RDI. Note the interesting comparison with two of the most popular diet plans of recent years.

Percentage of Recommended Daily Intake

Pritikin ☐   Fit For Life ▨   Fat or Fiction ■

17
DEALING WITH PEER PRESSURE

When you make positive changes in your eating and exercise regime you will be almost certain to encounter peer pressure. This may come from friends, family or work colleagues. When they begin to notice that you are choosing different foods from a menu, or starting to bring lunch from home, the questions will begin. This curiosity may evolve into lectures or challenges on the subject of diet. There is always someone who knows better.

Others will try to sabotage your efforts to change. Usually they want to justify why they are not making an effort to improve themselves. People will often make themselves feel better by ensuring that you are not going to outshine them. They feel guilty eating that sugar-laden dessert after dinner when you have no intention of joining them! We've all heard: 'Go on, just have a little bit', 'One won't do you any harm!', 'You only live once'.

Some words of advice:

- Be strong – don't allow others' insecurities to hinder your ability to make positive changes.
- Be a leader, not a follower. Don't be afraid to be different … you don't have to do the same as everyone else, just to 'fit in'.
- Try not to be evangelistic. If you try to 'convert' others because you are so enthusiastic about your new regime, no matter how genuine your intentions, this is asking for peer pressure! When the results are evident for all to see, you will be fighting off the hoards who will be begging for your secret!
- Be patient with yourself.
- Above all else, make the commitment and stick with it. The results will be more than worth it!

18
CONCLUSION

It's up to you!

At this point, you really need only ask yourself one question: 'Is what I am currently doing working for me?' If the answer is yes, then I doubt very much you would be reading this book. If the answer is no, then I suggest you try the approach that is offered here, even if it may conflict with some of your current beliefs.

If you can be sufficiently open-minded to try a change – and it is probably a radical change for many – you will find yourself pleasantly surprised. Whether your goal is to trim off some body fat, increase strength or endurance for sports conditioning, or to take control of ailments such as diabetes or high cholesterol problems, it is up to you.

I repeat, if you are currently taking any medication for existing ailments, please consult your physician before commencing any dramatic changes in your daily regimen, whether exercise, diet or both. When your health and fitness improve, you can give your doctor some advice!

If you find the idea of weighing and calculating your foods a waste of time and energy, then I suggest you do not even attempt to. This will cloud your efforts with a negative association and will soon become a chore that you will eliminate anyway. As a very simple rule, if you eat the foods suggested within the basic food listings provided, allowing your hunger to dictate the rest, you will achieve results. I have structured a basic menu outline to enable you to develop a sensible, nutritionally-balanced eating format that is flexible enough to last you a lifetime.

After all, the 'secret' to weight control is finding a program that you are comfortable to follow for the rest of your life, to maintain a healthy, disease-free body and optimum quality of life. So really, the secret is … that there is no secret!

Get started!

19
REFERENCES

Ascherio, A., Rimm, E.B., Stampfer, M.J., Giovannucci, E, L., Willett, W.C. Dietary intake of marine omega–3 fatty acids, fish intake, and the risk of coronary disease among men – *NEJM*. 332:977, 1995.

Atal S. The effects of dietary trans fatty acids on adipose composition and metabolism in male mice. C57B1/6J. College Park MD: Doctoral Dissertation, University of Maryland, 1990.

Australian Bureau of Statistics: *Australia's Food and Nutrition*, 1994.

Australian Bureau of Statistics: Health in Australia – what you should know, 1995.

Australian Bureau of Statistics: Apparent Consumption of Foodstuffs. 4306.0, 1996–97

Australian Bureau of Statistics: National Nutrition Survey, 4804.0 – Foods Eaten, Australia, 1995

Barbirol, B. et al. Genetic defects leading to muscle myopathies, *Journal of Neurology* (242:472–7). 1995.

Bendich, A.Safety issues regarding the use of vitamin supplements, *NY Academy Science*. 669:300–8. 1992

Bendich, A. and Langseth, L. Safety of Vitamin A. *American Journal Clinical Nutrition*, 49:358–71 1989

Bendich, Dr A. and. Passwater, Dr R. Vitamins, Immune response and safety, *Health World Online*, 15 Dec 98.

Berkson, B. *The Alpha Lipoic Acid Breakthrough*. 58–62, 1998

Bland, J.S. The changing nature or dietary fats and oils. *Let's Live*, 68–69. November 1987.

Bushkin, G. and E. *ALA Fights Free Radical Damage*. CNC. 1997.

Brown, M.S. and Goldstein, J.L. Atherosclerosis: Scavenging for receptors. *Nature* 343 (6258):506–9. 8 Feb. 1990.

Califano, J.A. What's wrong with U.S. health care? *Washington Post*, 26 June 1977.

Charles, Dr A.and Passwater, Dr R.A. *Measuring your Antioxidant*

Status; Clark, Dr J. and Passwater, Dr R.A. Lipoic Acid Basics Health.

Conte, Dr A. America's No. 1 Health Problem: Overweight but Undernourished; *Health World Online*, Dec. 98.

Dieber–Rotheneder, M., Puhl, H., Waeg, G., and Esterbauer, H.J. Lipid effect of oral supplementation with D–alpha–tocopherol on the vitamin E content of human low–density lipoproteins and resistance to oxidation. *Res*. 32:1325–32. 1991.

Enig, M.G. *Trans Fatty Acids in the Food Supply: A comprehensive report covering 60 years of research*, Silver Spring, MD: Enig Assoc., 1993.

Enig, M.G., Munn, R.J. and Keeney, M. Dietary Fat and Cancer Trends. A critique. *Federation Proceedings* 1978. 37:2215–2220.

Enig, Dr M. and Passwater, Dr R.A. Health Risks from Processed Foods and Trans Fats (Part 1 & 2) *Health World Online*, Dec. 98

Erasmus, U. *Fats and Oils*, Alive Books, Vancouver, 1986.

Esterbauer, Dr H. and Passwater, Dr R.A. Vitamin E and Carotenoids Protect Arteries from Cholesterol Deposits. *Health World Online*, Dec. 98.

Gaziano, J.M., Manson, J.E., Buring, J.E. and Hennekens, C.H. Dietary antioxidants and cardiovascular disease, Ann. *NY Academy Science* 1993. 249–59.

Halliwell, B., Gutteridge, J.M.C., Packer, L. and Glazer, A.N. Role of free radicals and catalytic metal ions in human disease: An overview. *Methods in Enzymology*, vol. 186, pp. 1–85, Academic Press, San Diego, 1990.

Harman, Dr D. and Passwater, Dr R.A. The Free Radical theory of Ageing (Part 1 & 2). *Health World Online*, Dec. 98.

Hennekens, Dr C. Improving the Health of the Public – Antioxidants and Heart Disease, *Health World Online*, Dec. 98.

Kirschmann, G.J. and Kirschmann, J.D. *Nutrition Almanac*, Nutrition Search Inc., 1996.

Langer, Dr S. 10 Antioxidants You Can Trust, *Better Nutrition Magazine*, May 98.

Leonard, R.E. Icons of American Diet Crash Into New Reality, *Nutrition Week*, 9 October 1992.

Mensink, R.P., Zock P.L., Katan, M.B. and Hornstra, G. Effect of dietary cis and trans fatty acids on serum lipoprotein [a] levels in humans, *J Lipid Res* 1992. 33: 1493 – 1501.

'McDonald's Should Revert to Old Fries', says CNI. *Nutrition Week* 1993; 23 (May 28):3 – anonymous.

Nutrition Research Newsletter. Fish oils and colon cancer (Diet & Cancer). Nov–Dec. 1992.11:126.

Packer, Dr L. *Free Radical Biology & Medicine*. (1995;19:227–50)

April, 1996 (FRBM; 20:625–6)

Packer, L. and Passwater, R.A.Oxygen radicals, Pro–oxidants and Antioxidant Nutrients, *Health World Online*, Dec. 98.

Passwater, RA. *Lipoic Acid – The Metabolic Antioxidant*. 1995.

Pauling, L. *How To Live Longer and Feel Better*. New York: W.H. Freeman & Co., 1986.

Pryor, Dr W. and Passwater, Dr R.A. Speaking of Radicals (Parts 1, 2 & 3). *Health World Online*, Dec. 1998.

Whiteman, M. et al., *FEBS Letters*, 1996. (379:74–6).

Willett, W.C., Stampfer, M.J., Manson, J.E., et al. Intake of trans fatty acids and risk of coronary heart disease among women. *The Lancet* 1993. (341:581–585).

EAT YOUR HEART OUT

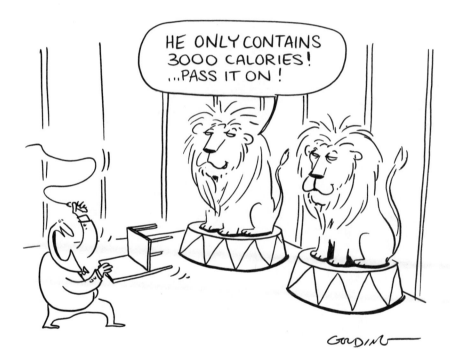

All nutritional calculations are approximate and will vary according to the ingredients used.

20
BREAKFAST

BREAKFAST SOUFFLE

Ingredients

6 egg whites
1 tablespoon protein powder
dash of vanilla essence
1 dessertspoon desiccated coconut

Method

Place egg whites in a mixing bowl and whip with electric mixer until thick peaks form, resembling meringue. Gradually add protein powder and vanilla essence, beating through thoroughly. Fold in coconut and spoon mixture into a bowl (approx. $^3/_4$ full to allow for rise). Place uncovered, into the microwave oven on medium heat for approximately 3 minutes, or until the soufflé rises and splits.

Note: If even slightly over-cooked, the texture will be heavy and rubbery.

Serve immediately sprinkled with Equal sweetener and cinnamon.

Calories: 160
Protein: 30 g
Carbohydrates: 1 g
Fat: 3 g
Fibre: 1 g

QUICK AND EASY OMELETTE

Ingredients

1 whole egg, 3 egg whites – beaten until light and fluffy
50 g lean ham or turkey, finely chopped
1 tablespoon grated cheese (i.e. parmesan, mozzarella, edam)
Dash of Tabasco sauce
Cracked pepper to taste
1 medium tomato
2 button mushrooms, diced

Method

Using a small, non-stick fry pan sprayed with oil, sauté ham/turkey, mushrooms and Tabasco sauce until thoroughly warmed through. Pour egg mixture over the top. Allow to set, using a spatula to tilt the liquid egg to the edges of the pan. When completely set, sprinkle the surface with cheese and use an egg-flip to fold in half.

Grind fresh black pepper over the top and serve with sliced, fresh or grilled tomato.

Calories: 215
Protein: 28 g
Carbohydrates: 5 g
Fat: 9 g
Fibre: 3.5 g

THICKSHAKES

Berry Delight

50 g frozen raspberries (no added sugar)
250 mL cold water
40 g (3 tablespoons) protein powder (low carbohydrate)
1 dessertspoon or 2 sachets of sweetener (e.g. Equal, Splenda)
10 mL 'Omega 3 and 6' oil (blend of safflower and flaxseed oils)
Place all ingredients in a blender. Blend until thoroughly combined.
Add extra water to alter thickness and texture if desired.

Serve immediately.

Calories: 254
Protein: 31 g
Carbohydrates: 10 g
Fat: 10 g
Fibre: 4 g

Mocha Supreme

200 mL cold water
1 cup crushed ice
1 teaspoon instant coffee, dissolved in 100 mL of boiling water,
cooled
2 teaspoons cocoa powder (unsweetened)
3 tablespoons protein powder (40 g)
1-2 dessertspoons of sweetener (Equal or Splenda)-to taste
1 heaped teaspoon psyllium husks
Blend all ingredients until combined. Serve immediately.

Caloriess: 167
Protein: 31 g
Carbohydrates: 5 g
Fat: 2.5 g
Fibre: 4 g

Vanilla Cinnamon Smoothie

1 teaspoon vanilla essence
200 mL cold water
1 cup crushed ice
3 tablespoons protein powder (40 g)
pinch of ground cinnamon to taste
1–2 dessertspoons of sweetener (Equal or Splenda) – to taste
1 heaped teaspoon psyllium husks
Blend all ingredients until combined. Serve immediately.

Calories: 154
Protein: 3 g
Carbohydrates: 3 g
Fat: 2 g
Fibre: 4 g

SAVORY EGGS AND CHEESE

Ingredients

1 whole egg, 3 egg whites, 30 g of grated cheese – beat until fluffy
Sprig of fresh, chopped parsley
Season-all spice, to taste
Serve with 1 grilled tomato

Method

Pour egg mixture into a preheated, non-stick pan sprayed with oil. Cook on a reasonably high heat and stir constantly to ensure the egg cooks evenly without browning. Add spice and parsley. When almost set, remove from the pan and serve immediately. Garnish with freshly ground, black pepper.

Calories: 155
Protein: 20 g
Carbohydrates: 1 g
Fat: 8 g
Fibre: 2 g

POACHED EGGS AND TOMATO

Ingredients

1 small tomato
2 whole eggs
1 tablespoon grated Parmesan cheese

Method

Fill a frypan with water approximately 3 cm deep and bring to the boil. To poach eggs, you may choose to use egg rings or add vinegar to the water to hold the eggs together. Add eggs to pan and simmer for approximately 3 minutes, or until appropriately set. Place tomato halves on a grill plate or pan sprayed with oil and allow to cook through and brown. Serve eggs and tomato immediately, sprinkle with grated cheese, cracked black pepper, or alternative seasoning, to taste.

Calories: 210
Protein: 16 g
Carbohydrates: 5 g
Fat: 14 g
Fibre: 2 g

BREAKFAST SAUSAGE

Ingredients

450 g lean, minced pork
1 teaspoon 'No Salt' (low sodium salt)
$^1/_2$ teaspoon black pepper
$^1/_2$ teaspoon sage
1 teaspoon onion powder
2 tablespoons wheat bran

Method

In a large mixing bowl, combine all ingredients and mix thoroughly. Refrigerate for 2 hours, then separate into 4 patties and cook over medium heat until well done.

Per serving

Calories: 160
Protein: 23 g
Carbohydrates: 0.5 g
Fat: 7 g
Fibre: 0.75 g

'LEGAL' PANCAKES

Ingredients

$^1/_4$ cup soy flour
$^1/_2$ cup protein powder (no added sugar)
$^1/_4$ cup almond meal
3 eggs
50 mL skim milk
1 tablespoon Splenda sweetener (or equivalent). Omit if savory topping is preferred
1 teaspoon baking powder

Method

Blend all ingredients in a blender or with electric mixer. Cook in a non-stick frypan sprayed lightly with oil, over medium heat. Brown on both sides.

Serving suggestions:

sugar-free maple syrup and fresh strawberries

low-carb. icecream and chopped nuts

Makes approx. 10 pancakes.

Per pancake (plain)

Calories: 78
Protein: 8.5 g
Carbohydrates: 1.6 g
Fat: 4.2 g
Fibre: 1 g

JAPANESE OMELETTE

Note: You will need a small non-stick rectangular fry pan to make this recipe. These pans are usually available from Asian grocers.

Ingredients

5 eggs
pinch of salt and pepper to season
1 level dessertspoon of cornstarch
olive oil (in a spray bottle or use a pastry brush)

Method

In a mixing bowl, combine all ingredients except the olive oil and whisk until combined, but not too frothy.

Lightly spray or brush the pan with oil and heat over a medium hotplate. Gently pour just enough of the egg mixture into the pan, to cover the entire surface with a paper-thin layer. Allow to set, tilting pan to ensure a very even coverage. At one end of the pan, gently lift the edge of the omelette with an egg flip and begin to form a tight roll, gradually rolling the mixture the full length of the pan. Push the roll back to the other end of the pan, pour in more mixture in a paper-thin layer, allow to set and repeat. (You may need to re-oil the pan between layers.) Continue this procedure until all egg mixture is used. Set aside the omelette and slice into round pieces, approximately 2 cm thick. This dish may be served hot or cold. Arrange on a serving platter with a small dish of soy sauce in the centre for dipping. Japanese omelette makes a tasty accompaniment to sashimi.

Note: As you become more confident with this recipe, you may experiment with fillings by adding very thin layers of deli meats, cheeses or grated vegetables during the rolling process.

To reduce the calories in this dish, remove 2 of the 5 whole eggs and replace with 4 extra egg whites.

Makes approx. 5 pieces (varying due to size of pan used)

Nutritional value per piece (without filling)

Calories: 90   Fat: 6 g
Protein: 6.5 g   Fibre: 0 g
Carbohydrates: 2.5 g

21
BISCUITS AND SNACKS

COCONUT MACAROONS

Ingredients

50 g almond meal
50 g unsweetened coconut
$1/_4$ teaspoon almond essence (optional)
1 teaspoon vanilla essence
pinch of salt
2 large egg whites
10g (1/2 cup) Splenda sweetener (or equivalent)

Method

Preheat oven to 300/150 degrees. Place almond meal, coconut, vanilla and almond essences in a large bowl. In a separate bowl beat egg whites and salt until stiff, then fold the dry ingredients through until thoroughly combined. Place teaspoon-sized balls of mixture onto a greased baking sheet. Bake for 25–30 minutes, or until lightly browned on the outside and soft on the inside.

Makes approx. 15 macaroons.

Per macaroon

Calories: 44
Protein: 1.2 g
Carbohydrates: 1.5 g
Fat: 3.7 g
Fibre: 1 g

BACON AND CHEESE BALLS

Ingredients

$^{1}/_{2}$ cup (60g) grated cheddar cheese
$^{1}/_{2}$ tablespoon of light mayonnaise
4 rashers of lean bacon, cooked until crisp, and crumbled

Method

Place all ingredients in a large bowl or blender and beat until combined. Form into 6 balls and store in airtight container in the refrigerator.

Calories: 100
Protein: 8 g
Carbohydrates: 1 g
Fat: 7 g
Fibre: 0 g

HI-FIBRE SLICE

Ingredients

80g dried apricots
80g raisins
50g desiccated coconut (unsweetened)
150g rolled oats
100g soy powder
4 egg whites
4 dessertspoons Splenda (or equivalent)
4 tablespoons tahini or nut paste
4 tablespoons sugarless jam
150 mL MCT oil (or 100 mL of unrefined, 'high oleic' oil)
80g protein powder (no added sugars)
250 mL flavored yogurt (no sugar added)
$^1/_2$ teaspoon cinnamon
50 g finely diced almonds

Method

Mix together all dry ingredients. In another large bowl, combine remaining ingredients and mix thoroughly. Gradually add dry ingredients until evenly distributed.

Scoop mixture into 5 rectangular, slice containers (approx. 12 cm x 7 cm) or one large, shallow, non-stick, baking pan.

Bake at 400 degrees for approx. 25–30 minutes.

Divided into 10 servings, per serve

Calories: 355
Protein: 20 g
Carbohydrates: 22 g
Fat: 20.5 g
Fibre: 5.8 g

*Note: This slice is higher in carbohydrates than most other recipes in this book, however, it is still in the range of 25% of the calories supplied by carbohydrate.

Be sure to consume this slice in moderation and take the carbohydrate content into account with your daily allowance.

CHOCOLATE FUDGE-BALLS

Ingredients

100 g protein powder (no added sugars)
50 g almond meal
50 g desiccated coconut (unsweetened)
1 heaped tablespoon tahini paste or nut paste
50 g cocoa (unsweetened)
50 g Equal sweetener
Cold water

Method

Combine all ingredients except water in a large bowl. Knead together into a paste, gradually adding cold water in small quantities, until it resembles a sticky, dough-like consistency.

Mould small balls and roll in additional coconut until thoroughly coated. Refrigerate. (Makes approximately 20 balls)

Approx. nutritional value per serve (average 20 serves)

Calories: 64
Protein: 5.5 g
Carbohydrates: 1.5 g
Fat: 4 g
Fibre: 0.65 g

RASPBERRY FUDGE-BALLS

Ingredients

100 g protein powder (no added sugars)
50 g almond meal
50 g desiccated coconut (unsweetened)
1 heaped tablespoon tahini paste or nut paste
1 punnet of fresh raspberries, pureed
50 g Equal sweetener

Method

Combine all ingredients in a large bowl. Mix thoroughly to form a sticky paste. A small quantity of cold water can be added to the mixture if it is too dry. Mould balls and roll in additional coconut until thoroughly coated. Refrigerate. (Makes approximately 20 balls)

Approx. nutritional value per serve (average 20 serves)

Calories: 60
Protein: 5.5 g
Carbohydrates: 1.5 g
Fat: 3.5 g
Fibre: .8 g

ANZAC BISCUITS

(makes approx. 10 biscuits)

Ingredients

$^1/_4$ cup almond meal
$^1/_4$ cup soy flour
$^1/_2$ cup rolled oats
$^1/_2$ cup desiccated coconut
$^1/_2$ cup Splenda sweetener
$^1/_4$ cup melted butter
2 tablespoons of 'sugar-free' maple syrup
$^1/_2$ teaspoon baking powder

Method

Preheat oven to 375 degrees. Grease a baking tray. In a large bowl, combine all dry ingredients. Melt the butter and pour into the mixture, along with the maple syrup. Stir until mixture is well combined. Form into dessertspoon-sized portions (make biscuits approx. 1 cm thick and 5 cm in diameter) and place on the baking tray. Cook in a moderately hot oven (375 degrees) for 18–22 minutes, or until biscuits are lightly browned.

Note: These biscuits are a carbohydrate-modified version of the original Anzac recipes. The carbohydrate content is still higher than the ideal, however, they are sugarless and contain more fibre and less carbohydrates than the regular recipes. They are intended as an occasional treat!

Approx. nutritional value per biscuit

Calories: 120
Protein: 2 g
Carbohydrates: 5.5 g
Fat: 10 g
Fibre: 1.8 gm

CHOCOLATE BISCUITS

Ingredients

100 g protein powder (no added sugar)
50 g almond meal
50 g desiccated coconut (unsweetened)
1 heaped tablespoon tahini paste or nut paste
50 g cocoa (unsweetened)
50 g sweetener (i.e. Splenda or equivalent) *
Cold water
*Must be a low-carbohydrate sweetener suitable for baking

Method

Combine all ingredients except water in a large bowl. Knead together into a paste, gradually adding cold water in small quantities until it resembles a sticky, dough-like consistency. (If using a liquid form of sweetener, use in place of water during mixing).

Roll biscuit dough on a flat, dry surface until as thin as possible. Use a biscuit cutter to form shape and bake on a nonstick tray or wax paper for approx. 20 minutes, or until crisp.

Remove from tray and cool. Store in an airtight container.

Makes approx. 40 biscuits, nutritional values per biscuit

Calories: 35
Protein: 2.8 g
Carbohydrates: .75 g
Fat: 2 g
Fibre: 0.35 g

22
SALADS

GREEK SALAD

Serves 4

Ingredients

Approx. 200 g lettuce leaves, torn into bite-size pieces
1 small, Spanish onion, sliced and separated into rings
150g Fetta cheese, cubed
Approx. 12 fresh, black olives, drained
1 large tomato, cut into bite-size wedges
1 medium cucumber, thinly sliced
$^1/_2$ green capsicum, cut into thin strips (julienne)
Dressing: 100 mL light, virgin, olive oil
100 mL vinegar (regular or balsamic)
juice of 1 lemon
(A commercial brand of vinaigrette, without sugar added, may
be substituted for the dressing)

Method

Place all ingredients in a large salad bowl. Mix together dressing ingredients and pour over salad, toss thoroughly and serve immediately.

Note: Do not add dressing until ready to serve.

Per serve

With dressing:	*Without dressing:*
Calories: 390	Calories: 170
Protein: 7 g	Protein: 7 g
Carbohydrates: 7.5 g	Carbohydrates: 7.5 g
Fat: 37 g	Fat: 12.5 g
Fibre: 4.5 g	Fibre: 4.5 g

Serve as a side dish with steak, chicken or fish.

TASTY 'CAESAR – STYLE' SALAD

Serves 6

Ingredients

2 large cos lettuces
2 tablespoons shaved, fresh Parmesan cheese
2 rashers of lean bacon, diced and dry fried (drain on paper towel)
1 medium tomato, finely diced
6-8 anchovy fillets, drained (optional)
2 hard-boiled eggs
Commercial Caesar dressing – approx. 2 tablespoons (low oil and sugar free)

Method

Tear lettuce into bite-sized pieces and place in a large salad bowl. Add Parmesan, cooled bacon, tomato, eggs and anchovy fillets. Toss with desired amount of dressing prior to serving.

Note: This salad can make a delicious lunch or a complete meal with the addition of extra protein, e.g., grilled chicken breast slices, sliced/shaved ham or turkey breast, tuna, sliced steak. It can be served with a warm poached egg on top instead of the hard-boiled egg mixed into the greens.

Approx. nutritional values per serving – 1/6 salad with anchovies (without addition of extra protein)

Calories: 165
Protein: 11.25 g
Carbohydrates: 2.5 g
Fats: 12.25 g
Fibre: .25 g

CHEF'S SALAD

Serves 4

Ingredients

2 heads of lettuce (any variety) – torn into bite-sized pieces
1 large tomato, diced
1 cucumber, diced
4 hard-boiled eggs (cut into halves)
200g cooked chicken breast (cut into strips)
200g sliced ham (cut into strips)
150g cheddar or Swiss cheese (julienne strips or grated)
Dressing: 2 tablespoons balsamic vinegar, 2 tablespoons
flaxseed oil, juice of 1 lemon; or 4 tablespoons of 'light' or 'free'
French dressing (low oil, no added sugar)

Method

Place lettuce, cucumber and tomato in a large salad bowl. Add dressing and toss until evenly distributed. Arrange eggs, chicken, ham and cheese on the top of the salad, serve immediately.

(If making salad in advance, add dressing and remaining ingredients just prior to serving time.)

Per serve

Calories: 315
Protein: 35 g
Carbohydrates: 5 g
Fat: 17 g
Fibre: 3 g

23
STARTERS

VEGETABLE SOUP

Serves 6

Ingredients

1 tablespoon virgin olive oil
1 medium onion, diced
2 small carrots, diced
2 medium parsnips or equivalent amount of pumpkin, diced
$^1/_2$ medium cabbage, shredded
2 large tomatoes, peeled and roughly diced
$^1/_2$ teaspoon Season-all spice
1 tablespoon Worcestershire sauce
1 tablespoon 'light' ketchup
1 tablespoon cornstarch (dissolved in water)
approx. 1.5 litres of clear stock/broth

Method

Heat oil in large stockpot, add onion and bacon and soften, stirring continuously. Add remaining ingredients, bring to the boil, then reduce to a simmer, covered with a lid, for approximately one hour.

Soup may be reheated as required, and/or frozen in required serving quantities.

Nutritional value per serve

Calories: 103
Protein: 5 g
Carbohydrates: 13 g
Fat: 3.5 g
Fibre: 3.6 g

Note: Any vegetables may be used in this soup apart from the obviously high starch variety.

Calories and other nutritional information above are approximate and will vary due to vegetable selection.

Note: To add carbohydrate-free ' noodles' to your soup, try making a thin omelette with eggs and a small amount of cornstarch to hold it together. When cooked and cooled, cut into length-wise strips and add to soup before reheating to serve.

PRAWN COCKTAIL

Serves 4

Ingredients

16 chilled, king prawns (cooked, de-veined and heads removed)
2 cups of shredded iceberg lettuce
1 lemon cut into 4 wedges (garnish)
Sauce:
4 tablespoons of 'light' mayonnaise
1 tablespoon tomato ketchup
2 teaspoons soy sauce
juice of 1 small lemon
Mix together until thoroughly blended, chill in refrigerator until ready to serve.

Method

Place shredded lettuce in 4 small glass serving bowls. Arrange 4 prawns around the edges of each bowl. Spoon over cocktail sauce and garnish with lemon wedges.

(Alternatively, baby shrimp or a combination of other shellfish meat (i.e. crab), may be used. Toss fish in sauce and serve over bed of chilled lettuce.

Per serve, king prawns

Calories: 130
Protein: 14 g
Carbohydrates: 12 g
Fat: 2 g
Fibre: 1 g

HAM AND MELON

Serves 4

Ingredients

1 small (400g) cantaloupe
8 very thin slices of Prosciutto or regular deli-cut ham

Method

Cut melon into 8 wedges and carefully remove seeds. Wrap a slice of prosciutto around each melon wedge, chill and serve as a snack or starter to a meal.

Per serve (2 wedges)

Calories: 95
Protein: 11 g
Carbohydrates: 7.5 g
Fat: 2.5 g
Fibre: 1.5 g
Nutritional values vary depending on ham used.

STUFFED 'ITALIAN' PEPPERS

Serves 2

Ingredients

2 large red or green capsicum
150 g of lean minced turkey, chicken or beef, cooked through
and drained of excess juices. Tinned tuna may be used (200g)
1 small, Spanish (red) onion, finely minced
$^1/_2$ teaspoon dried oregano
$^1/_2$ teaspoon dried basil
1 fresh garlic clove, crushed (optional)
30 g 'light' mozzarella or cheddar cheese, grated
1 tablespoon Parmesan cheese, grated
1 tablespoon spicy tomato-based pasta sauce (no added sugar)

Method

Preheat oven to 350 degrees. Slice off the tops of the capsicum and set aside. Remove the core, seeds and white inner 'seams' of the capsicum. Mix together all remaining ingredients, except cheeses. Before filling them, make sure the bottom of the capsicum are even enough to stand on the baking tray. Trim where necessary for stability. Spoon filling into the peppers, add the 'lids' and place them in a shallow baking tray with $^1/_2$ cup of water. Bake for approximately 30 minutes, or until tender. Remove lids and heap cheeses on top. Return to the oven until cheese has melted. Serve with a green salad or coleslaw.

Per pepper: (will vary according to meat selection)

Calories: 205
Protein: 24 g
Carbohydrates: 11.5 g
Fat: 7 g
Fibre: 3.5 g

24
MAIN MEALS

CHICKEN STIR-FRY

Serves 4

Ingredients

3 large chicken breast fillets (skin removed), cut into thin strips
(may substitute with lean beef, pork or fish fillets)
1 cup broccoli pieces
1 cup cauliflower pieces
1 cup snow peas or 1 red capsicum (sliced into strips)
1 carrot, julienned
$^1/_2$ medium onion
$^1/_2$ small cabbage (or equivalent in bok choy), finely shredded
2 tablespoons soy sauce
1 tablespoon 'light' tomato ketchup
juice of 1 lemon
Season-all spice, to taste
1 tablespoon sesame seeds
1 clove freshly ground garlic (optional)
2 tablespoons of oil (i.e. 'high oleic', safflower/sunflower oil or
virgin olive oil)

Method

Heat oil in a large, deep non-stick pan or wok. Sauté onion and garlic until softened. Add chicken pieces and cook through, constantly stirring. Add all remaining ingredients and turn to a low heat, simmering with a lid until vegetables are cooked to desired tenderness. (Take care not to over-cook, ideally vegetables should remain slightly crispy.)

Serve immediately with shaved or grated Parmesan cheese.

Approx. nutritional value per serving

Calories: 263
Protein: 27 g
Carbohydrates: 9.5 g
Fat: 13 g
Fibre: 5 g

SALMON CAKES

Serves 4

Ingredients

300g tinned red salmon (drained)
1 cup of diced fresh pumpkin (cooked and pureed until smooth)
1 small onion, finely grated
$^1/_2$ teaspoon Season-all spice
1 tablespoon of hot taco salsa (no added sugar)
30g almond meal
2 tablespoons of grated Parmesan cheese

Method

Place all ingredients into a large mixing bowl. Mix thoroughly and mould into small patties (approx. 2 tablespoons of mixture per patty). Refrigerate for several hours to set. Salmon cakes may be grilled until brown and warmed through, or cooked in a small amount of oil in a fry pan.

Serve hot or cold with salad of your choice.

Per serving (no added fat for cooking):

Calories: 200
Protein: 20.5 g
Carbohydrates: 5 g
Fat: 11 g
Fibre: 2.5 g

BARBEQUE KEBABS

Serves 4

Ingredients

300g of cubed chicken breast, lean beef, lamb or pork
2 medium onions, cut into 16 wedges
1 red and 1 green capsicum, cut into squares (approx. 3 cm sq.)
8 small cherry tomatoes
4 rashers of bacon (optional) – cut into 3 cm-square pieces
8 steel or wooden skewers (approx. 20-30 cm long)
Marinade: 4 tablespoons of 'high oleic' safflower oil or virgin olive oil
2 tablespoons of Worcestershire sauce
juice of 1 lemon
Season-all spice

Method

Place on the skewers, in any sequence,3 cubes of meat, 2 onion wedges, capsicum in each color, a cherry tomato, and 2 pieces of bacon.

Prepare 8 skewers, place in a large flat dish side by side, sprinkle with spice and pour over marinade. Leave for 4 hours or overnight before cooking. Place on a barbeque or grill tray and cook until meat is evenly done, basting with remaining marinade during cooking time.

Note: Take care not to place ingredients too close to each other on skewers, to ensure even cooking.

Serve with your favorite salad or vegetables.

Serving per 2 skewers, approx. (variation due to meat used)

Without bacon:	*With bacon:*
Calories: 245	Calories: 345
Protein: 10.5 g	Protein: 18.5 g
Carbohydrates: 5.5 g	Carbohydrates: 5.5 g
Fat: 20 g	Fat: 28 g
Fibre: 2.5 g	Fibre: 2.5 g

ITALIAN STYLE MEATBALLS

(makes approximately 10 meatballs)

Ingredients

500 g lean, ground beef
$^1/_2$ medium onion, finely diced
1 clove fresh garlic (optional)
1 tablespoon sugar-free tomato paste
1 egg, beaten
$^1/_2$ cup water
2 tablespoons virgin olive oil
salt and pepper to taste
1 tablespoon wheat bran
2 tablespoons almond meal

Method

In a large mixing bowl, combine all ingredients except oil and mix until thoroughly blended. Mould into approx. 10 meatballs and refrigerate for a minimum of 1 hour.

Heat oil in non-stick frypan and toss meatballs over medium heat until lightly browned and cooked through.

Per meatball

Calories: 132
Protein: 11.5 g
Carbohydrates: 1.4 g
Fat: 8.9 g
Fibre: 2 g

CHICKEN CORDON BLEU

Serves 4

Ingredients

2 large chicken breast fillets (skin and bone removed)
$^1/_4$ teaspoon Season-all spice
2 eggs beaten lightly
4 thin slices of lean ham
4 thin slices of cheddar or Swiss cheese
1 cup chicken broth

Method

Preheat oven to 350 degrees.

Cut the breast fillets in half and pound with a mallet until as thin as possible. Sprinkle meat with Season-all spice. Place one piece of ham and a piece of cheese on top of each chicken breast, then roll each breast with ham and cheese inside.

Tie each roll with string to secure. Place rolls in a baking dish and pour over chicken broth.

Bake uncovered for approx. 1 hour.

Serve 1 roll to each person with a selection of fresh vegetables or salad.

Note: rolls may be refrigerated and sliced as a cold snack.

Per roll

Calories: 200
Protein: 29 g
Carbohydrates: 0 g
Fat: 10 g
Fibre: 0 g

HAMBURGERS

Serves 4

Ingredients

300 g lean minced beef
1 small onion, finely diced
$^1/_2$ teaspoon garlic powder (optional)
$^1/_2$ teaspoon barbeque seasoning
25 g almond meal
1 tablespoon Worcestershire sauce

Topping ingredients

2 button mushrooms, thinly sliced
4 slices of tasty cheese
$^1/_2$ tomato, cut into 4 thin slices

Method

In a large mixing bowl, combine all burger ingredients and mix thoroughly. Form into 4 round, flat burgers, approx. 2 cm thick. (If burgers are too thick, topping is difficult to place on top.) Refrigerate to set for a couple of hours or overnight. Grill or barbeque until browned and cooked through. In a lightly oiled non-stick pan, sauté mushrooms. Add mushrooms to the top of each burger, followed by a slice of tomato and cheese. Place under grill and cook until cheese has begun to melt. Serve with a tossed green salad or vegetables.

Per burger

Calories: 220
Protein: 22 g
Carbohydrates: 1.5 g
Fat: 14 g
Fibre: 1.2 g

MEAT AND VEGETABLE PASTIE

Serves 4

Ingredients

4 sheets of filo pastry
Filling
200 g lean beef mince
¹/₂ small onion, finely diced
¹/₂ green capsicum, finely diced
¹/₂ medium carrot, finely diced
¹/₂ cup green peas (80g)
olive oil (in spray bottle or use pastry brush)
2 tablespoons taco sauce (no added sugar)
¹/₂ medium tomato, finely diced
¹/₂ teaspoon Season-all spice
30 g sesame seeds

Method

Preheat oven to 375 degrees.

Spray a non-stick pan with oil, add onion, capsicum and carrot and cook until softened. Add beef and cook through. Add remaining filling ingredients and heat through until softened. To make filo parcels, lay out a pastry sheet on a flat, dry surface. Spray or brush with oil and fold the sheet lengthwise into 3 folds. At the top end of your long pastry strip, place a small amount of filling (approx. 2 tablespoons) and continue to fold down the strip to form a triangular parcel. Spray or brush the top with oil, sprinkle with sesame seeds and place on a greased tray (high oven shelf) for approx. 25 minutes, or until golden brown.

Remove and serve hot with a fresh green salad.

Approx. nutritional value per pastie

Calories: 190
Protein: 14 g
Carbohydrates: 14 g
Fat: 8.5 g
Fibre: 3 g

CHICKEN AND CHEESE PASTIE

Serves 4

Ingredients

4 sheets of filo pastry
Filling

1 medium, skinless, chicken breast fillet, cooked and finely diced
100g of frozen spinach, thawed and thoroughly drained
50 g 'light' ricotta cheese
$^1/_2$ cup broccoli, broken into tiny flowerets
1 tablespoon taco sauce
olive oil (in a spray bottle or use pastry brush)
30 g sesame seeds
Season-all spice

Method

Preheat oven to 375 degrees.

Lightly cook broccoli and spinach. Remove from heat and cool. Add chicken, cheese, taco sauce and spice, mix until evenly combined.

Lay out pastry sheet on a flat, dry surface. Spray or brush with oil and fold lengthwise into 3 folds. At the top end of your long pastry strip, place approx. 2 tablespoons of mixture and continue to fold down the strip to form a triangular parcel. Spray or brush the top with oil, sprinkle with sesame seeds and place on a greased tray (high oven shelf) for approx. 25 minutes or until lightly browned.

Remove and serve hot with a fresh green salad.

Approx. nutritional value per pastie

Calories: 145
Protein: 9.5 g
Carbohydrates: 12 g
Fat: 6.5 g
Fibre: 2.5 g

QUICHE LORRAINE

Serves 8

Ingredients

Pastry

2 tablespoons Parmesan cheese, grated
1 egg
20g softened butter
50g almond meal
25g sesame seeds
pinch of salt

Method

Place all ingredients in a large mixing bowl and beat until well combined. Lightly brush an ovenproof quiche dish with oil and press a thin, even layer of the mixture over the base and up the sides of the dish.

Filling

8 rashers of lean bacon (fat trimmed), diced and grilled
4 eggs
4 tablespoons of grated Parmesan cheese
30 g grated, light cheddar cheese
100 mL light cream
1 dessertspoon taco sauce (no added sugar)
$^1/_2$ medium onion, diced
$^1/_2$ teaspoon season – all spice
1 teaspoon dried parsley

Method

Sauté onion in a lightly oiled non-stick pan until transparent and softened; cool. In a large mixing bowl, combine all ingredients and mix thoroughly.

Pour into pastry shell and cook in a preheated oven to 350 degrees for approx. 30 minutes, or until filling is set and lightly browned. Serve hot or cold with your favorite salad or cut into small squares and present as hors d'oeuvres.

Serve with a tossed green salad.

Approx. nutritional value per 1/8 serving

With pastry:	*Without pastry:*
Calories: 206.5	Calories: 143
Protein: 16 g	Protein: 12 g
Carbohydrates: 0.6 g	Carbohydrates: 0.6 g
Fat: 16 g	Fat: 9.5 g
Fibre: 1 g	Fibre: .25 g

LASAGNE

Serves 8

Ingredients

500 g lean beef mince
1 medium onion, finely diced
1 clove garlic, crushed (optional)
1 375gm tin of diced tomatoes (no added sugar)
2 tablespoons tomato-based pasta sauce (no added sugar)
1 large carrot, finely diced
100 g fresh button mushrooms, diced
1 teaspoon dried oregano
1 teaspoon dried basil
1 large cabbage
150 g Parmesan cheese, grated
250 g mozzarella cheese, grated

Method

Sauté onion and garlic in a lightly-oiled, large pan, until softened. Add beef and cook until browned. Add tomatoes, pasta sauce, oregano, basil, mushroom and carrot. Bring to boil and reduce to a simmer for approx. 30 minutes.

Preheat oven to 350 degrees and lightly oil a large, rectangular baking dish. Gently remove the largest cabbage leaves keeping them intact (you will need enough leaves to cover your baking dish twice). Blanche cabbage in boiling water until softened, remove and place in iced water, then pat dry with paper towel.

Place a layer of meat sauce to cover the bottom of the baking dish (1/2 of total amount). Cover with a layer of cabbage leaves, then a layer of combined cheeses (1/2 total amount). Repeat layers and sprinkle remaining cheese over the top.

Place in oven (middle shelf) and cook for approx. 30 minutes, or until cheese is lightly browned and dish is cooked through.

Serve with a tossed green salad.

Nutritional value per 1/8 slice

Calories: 269
Protein: 28 g
Carbohydrates: 6.5 g
Fat: 14.5 g
Fibre: 2 g

VEGETABLE BOLOGNAISE

Serves 4

Ingredients

4 cups of mixed vegetables, fresh or frozen (julienned carrots, broccoli, cauliflower, snow peas, capsicum, cabbage, etc.)
Note: choose a colorful variety of approx. 4 different vegetables
250 g lean, minced beef
1 small onion, finely diced
1 clove garlic, crushed (optional)
$\frac{1}{2}$ large tin of diced tomatoes (no added sugar)
1 tablespoon tomato-based pasta sauce (no added sugar)
1 small carrot, finely diced
$\frac{1}{2}$ teaspoon dried oregano
$\frac{1}{2}$ teaspoon dried basil
Approx. 4 tablespoons fresh Parmesan cheese, grated or shaved

Method

Sauté onion and garlic in a lightly oiled pan until softened. Add beef and cook until browned. Add tomatoes, pasta sauce, carrot, oregano and basil. Bring to the boil, then simmer for 60 minutes, stirring occasionally.

Steam vegetables and arrange on 4 serving plates. Spoon meat sauce over the centre of the vegetables, as you would over a pasta dish. Sprinkle with a tablespoon of fresh, grated or shaved Parmesan, or place Parmesan in a small bowl at the table.

Per serve (including Parmesan cheese)

Calories: 160
Protein: 17.5 g
Carbohydrates: 7 g
Fat: 6.5 g
Fibre: 4.5 g

WORCESTERSHIRE CHICKEN

Serves 4

Ingredients

600 g chicken breast fillets – skinned and boned, diced into cubes
$^1/_2$ medium onion, finely diced
1 clove garlic, crushed (optional)
5 tablespoons Worcestershire sauce (lowest carb. avail.)
Juice of 1 large lemon
$^1/_4$ cup dry white wine
cracked black pepper, to taste
1 tablespoon wheat bran
2 tablespoons virgin olive oil for cooking
1 teaspoon Season-all spice

Method

In a large, non-stick skillet, fry onion and garlic in oil until softened. Add chicken and spice and toss until slightly browned. Add Worcestershire, lemon juice, wine and pepper, cover with a lid and bring to boil. Reduce heat to a simmer and cook for a further 30-40 minutes. Stir in wheat bran and allow to stand for 5 minutes. Serve with a tossed green salad or your favorite vegetables.

Per serving

Calories: 255
Protein: 20.5 g
Carbohydrates: 5 g
Fat: 17 g
Fibre: 1.1 g

CHICKEN AND BROCCOLI FRITTATA

Serves 4

Ingredients

6 whole eggs + 4 egg whites
100 mL evaporated skim milk (Carnation)
1 small onion, finely diced
pinch of salt and pepper
1 crushed clove of garlic (optional)
2 teaspoons wheat bran or flax powder
3 tablespoons grated Parmesan cheese
150 g chicken, cooked and cubed
50 g light cheddar cheese, grated
1 cup of fresh broccoli (small pieces)
olive oil (in a spray bottle or use a pastry brush)
1 tablespoon taco sauce (no added sugar)

Method

In a mixing bowl, combine all eggs, salt and pepper, milk and 2 of the 3 tablespoons of Parmesan cheese. Blend together with a whisk or electric mixer. In a lightly oiled pan, cook onion until transparent. Add chicken, broccoli and taco sauce to the pan and simmer until cooked through. Add wheat bran and stir until combined. Pour egg mixture over the pan ingredients and continue to cook over a low heat until egg is set. During cooking, tilt uncooked egg to the side of the pan to ensure even cooking. Sprinkle the remaining Parmesan and cheddar cheese over the top and place pan under a hot grill until cheese is browned and melted.

Cut into 4 wedges and serve with a tossed green salad.

Per serve

Calories: 270
Protein: 28.5 g
Carbohydrates: 7.5 g
Fat: 14 g
Fibre: 3.5 g

CHICKEN MEATBALLS

Serves 4

Ingredients

500g lean chicken mince (breast meat only)
1 egg, beaten
2 tblsp fresh, chopped basil
30 g almond meal
1 tblsp olive oil
20 g butter

Method

Combine chicken mince, egg, basil and almond meal and mix well. Divide mixture into 12 portions and roll into balls. Heat oil and butter and cook chicken balls until lightly browned on all sides. Allow to cook through.

Chicken meatballs may be served as a finger-food, or accompaniment to soups or stir-fried vegetables.

Note: meatballs may be frozen for up to 8 weeks.

Per serve

Calories: 267
Protein: 31.5 g
Carbohydrates: 0.3 g
Fat: 15.5 g
Fibre: 0.6 g

SALMON FRITTATA

Serves 4

Ingredients

6 whole eggs + 4 egg whites
100 mL evaporated skim milk (Carnation)
Pinch of salt and pepper
1 small onion, finely diced
2 teaspoons wheat bran
2 tablespoons grated Parmesan cheese
200 g red salmon, drained
50 g light cheddar cheese
1 tablespoon taco sauce (no added sugar)
olive oil (in a spray bottle or use a pastry brush)

Method

In a large mixing bowl, combine all eggs, milk, salt and pepper, salmon, taco sauce, 1 of the 2 tablespoons of parmesan cheese and wheat bran. Blend with electric mixer until thoroughly combined. In a non-stick pan sprayed or brushed with oil, sauté onions until transparent. Add egg mix to pan and simmer on low heat until set, tilting pan to allow uncooked mixture to run to the edges. When set, top with remaining parmesan and cheddar cheese, then place under a hot grill until cheese is lightly browned.

Cut into 4 wedges and serve with salad and seafood sauce.

Per serve (without sauce)

Calories: 298
Protein: 32 g
Carbohydrates: 3 g
Fat: 17 g
Fibre: 1.5 g

WIENER SCHNITZEL

Serves 4

Note: For this recipe you will need a meat mallet or rolling pin

Ingredients

*4 chicken breast or lean veal fillets, approx. 100 g each (skin
and bone removed)*
1 large egg, lightly beaten
1 teaspoon Season-all spice
50 g of almond meal
olive oil spray or use a pastry brush

Method

Place a sheet of waxed paper over chicken and pound or roll each
piece evenly until thin. Dip each fillet in egg and coat in combined
spice and almond meal until completely covered. Refrigerate for
at least 2 hours. Heat a large non-stick skillet sprayed with oil.
Place 'crumbed' meat in the heated pan and cook each side until
cooked through and lightly browned. Serve hot or cold with wedges
of fresh lemon and a tossed green salad.

Per fillet (will vary depending on meat used):

Calories: 269
Protein: 30 g
Carbohydrates: 1.2 g
Fat: 16 g
Fibre: 2.3 g

HAM AND VEGETABLE FRITTATA

Ingredients

150 g lean ham, roughly chopped
100 g light Mozzarella cheese, grated
10 eggs
¹/₂ teaspoon Tabasco sauce
1 tablespoon tomato paste or sugar-free tomato pasta sauce
1 cup of mixed chopped vegetables (e.g. broccoli, carrot,
zucchini)
1 small onion, finely diced
Season-all spice

Method

Preheat oven to 350/180 degrees. Grease a non-stick baking tin (approx. 20 cm square). In a non-stick frypan, sauté onions, ham, tomato paste, spice and vegetables until tender. Break eggs into a large bowl with half of the cheese and Tabasco sauce. Beat until combined. Place the ham and vegetable mixture into the prepared baking tin and spread evenly over the base. Pour egg mixture over the ham and vegetables and bake until set. (Mixture may need stirring during cooking time to ensure even cooking). Sprinkle remaining cheese over the top of the frittata and place under a grill until cheese is browned.

Cut into 10 wedges and serve hot or cold with your favorite salad.

Per serve

Calories: 129
Protein: 12 g
Carbohydrates: 1.7 g
Fat: 8.2 g
Fibre: 1 g
To reduce total calorie content, you may decrease the quantity of egg yolks and replace the volume with egg whites(e.g. 4 whole eggs and 10 whites).

25
DESSERTS

CHOCOLATE MOUSSE

6 servings

Ingredients

1 x 375mL tin of light evaporated milk – chilled (reserve tin to refill with cold water)
375 mL of cold water
150 g protein powder (pref. vanilla – no added sugar)
4–5 dessertspoons of Splenda sweetener
2 sachets of plain gelatin dissolved in 100 mL of boiling water (slightly cooled)
2 level dessertspoons of cocoa powder (or to taste)
4 egg whites (at room temperature)

Method

Pour the tin of milk into a large mixing bowl, refill tin with cold water and add to the milk. Using an electric beater, gradually add sweetener, followed by protein powder and cocoa. Beat until a thick and creamy consistency. In a separate bowl, beat the egg whites until stiff peaks form. Add dissolved gelatin to the milk mixture and continue to beat until thoroughly combined. Gently fold through egg whites and pour into airtight container/s. Refrigerate until set.

Alternatively, place in an airtight container/s in the freezer for a couple of hours to form ice-cream.

Per serve

Calories: 126
Protein: 18 g
Carbohydrates: 10 g
Fat: 1.5 g
Fibre: 0 g

BANANA MOUSSE

Serves 6

Ingredients

*1 x 375mL tin of light evaporated milk – chilled (reserve tin to
refill with cold water)*
375 mL of cold water
100 g protein powder (pref. vanilla)
*banana flavored, sugar-free jelly crystals (enough to make 1
litre of jelly), dissolved in 100 mL of boiling water (slightly
cooled)*
4 egg whites (at room temperature)

Method

Pour the tin of milk into a large mixing bowl, refill tin with cold
water and add to the milk. Using an electric beater, gradually add
protein powder until thick and creamy. In a separate bowl, beat
egg whites until stiff peaks form. To the milk mixture, add the
dissolved and slightly cooled jelly crystals and beat until combined.
Gently fold in egg whites. Pour into airtight container/s and
refrigerate until set.

Per serve

Calories: 121
Protein: 19 g
Carbohydrates: 9 g
Fat: 1 g
Fibre: 0 g

CHEESECAKE

Ingredients

Base

50 g almond meal
1 rounded tablespoon (30g) of tahini paste or nut butter (sugar-free)
30 g protein powder
100 g of butter, softened
50 g or 100 mL of artificial sweetener (suitable for baking)
50 g of desiccated coconut
$\frac{1}{4}$ teaspoon mixed spice or cinnamon
2 eggs

Method

Preheat oven to 350 degrees. Grease a large spring-form cake tin (approx. 25 cm diameter).

In a large bowl, beat together butter, tahini, eggs, sweetener and spice. Gradually add the remaining dry ingredients until thoroughly combined into a smooth paste. Spread the mixture over the base of the baking tin as thinly as possible. Bake until firm and slightly crispy. Allow to cool.

Filling
500 g of cream cheese (regular = 33% fat)
500 mL cream (full-fat or reduced)
100 g protein powder
250 g natural yogurt
juice and rind of one lemon*
dash of vanilla essence*
gelatin (1 sachet dissolved in 100 mL of boiling water)*
100 g of Splenda sweetener.

Method

Combine cream cheese, cream and yogurt. Beat with electric beater until combined and smooth. Gradually add sweetener and protein powder and continue to beat until smooth and creamy.

*At this point you can vary the flavor added by choosing lemon, vanilla and gelatin for vanilla flavor, or alternatively, divide the mixture in half and create 2 flavors.

Strawberry – omit lemon, vanilla, half the sweetener and gelatin, and replace with 1 sachet of 'diet' strawberry jelly crystals dissolved in 100 mL of boiling water.

Chocolate – omit lemon and vanilla, add approx. 2 tablespoons of unsweetened cocoa powder.

Add gelatin or jelly crystals last. If splitting mixture into two flavors, be sure to refrigerate and partially set the initial layer over the cooked base before adding gelatin to the second layer. When the first layer is set, continue to add the second layer over the top. When completed and set, you may decorate with whipped cream and fruit for serving.

Note: Calories and nutritional value will vary due to choice of flavor, as well as choice of full cream or low-fat cream and cheese. Total calories can be reduced by using 'light' cream cheese and reduced-fat cream (beware of additional carbohydrates). This is obviously not designed to be a low-calorie dessert, but the protein content is high and carbohydrates minimal, per serve.

Per serve ($^1/_{12}$ of total cheesecake)

Calories: 469
Protein: 14.5 g
Carbohydrates: 4.3 g
Fat: 43.7 g
Fibre: 1.5 g

FLAVORED PROTEIN – CREAM

Serves 4

Ingredients

200 mL thickened cream
3 sachets of Splenda sweetener (or equivalent)
2 dessertspoons protein powder (no carbohydrates)
Flavoring:
1 teaspoon vanilla/banana/strawberry or other essence

Method

Pour cream into a small mixing bowl. Add all remaining ingredients and whip with electric mixer until cream is thick and all ingredients blended thoroughly.

Serving suggestions:

Use to fill hi-fibre slice, serve with fresh strawberries or a small quantity of stewed apple.

Per serve

Calories: 205
Protein: 20 g
Carbohydrates: 0 g
Fat: 14 g
Fibre: 0 g

CHOCOLATE SPONGE CAKE

Ingredients

4 eggs, separated (at room temperature)
¹/₂ teaspoon cream of tartar
3 heaped tablespoons Splenda sweetener (or equivalent)
2 heaped tablespoon protein powder
25 g fine-ground almond meal
1 tablespoon of cocoa powder (unsweetened), sifted

Method

Preheat oven to 350 degrees and grease a cake tin.

In a mixing bowl, whip egg whites until they resemble meringue. Gradually add sweetener and continue beating until combined. In another bowl, sift together cocoa, protein powder, almond meal and cream of tartar. Beat yolks in a separate bowl, then fold into the egg-white mixture. Gradually add the sifted dry ingredients, gently folding through the egg mixture until combined, taking care not to break down the egg white. Pour mixture into the prepared cake tin and bake in a moderate oven for approximately 20–25 minutes, or until a cake tester can be inserted into the cake and removed clean.

Per serve (¹/₆ of cake)

Calories: 91.5
Protein: 7 g
Carbohydrates: 1 g
Fat: 8.5 g
Fibre: 0.5 g

26
MISCELLANEOUS

PARTY DIP

Ingredients

200 g light cottage cheese
200 g tin of tuna in water
dash of Tabasco sauce
1 heaped tablespoon of light mayonnaise
2 hard-boiled eggs, finely chopped
salt and pepper to taste

Method

Combine all ingredients and mix well. (Add Tabasco sauce to taste.)
Place in a small serving bowl and surround with a large platter of
fresh vegetable strips (e.g. carrots, celery, cucumber).

Approx. nutritional value per vegetable stick plus 1 scoop of dip

Calories: 30
Protein: 4 g
Carbohydrates: 2 g
Fat: 1 g
Fibre: 1 g

RASPBERRY JAM

Ingredients

300 g of frozen or fresh raspberries (no added sugar)
1 sachet of strawberry jelly crystals (sugar free) – to make
250 mL of jelly
250 mL of boiling water
1 teaspoon of raspberry or strawberry extract

Method

Defrost berries. Add boiling water to jelly crystals and stir until dissolved. Place jelly in refrigerator and cool until it begins to thicken, but not set completely. Boil or microwave berries for approx. 3–5 minutes. Remove from heat and cool. Add strawberry extract and fold berries into jelly mix. Mix thoroughly and refrigerate.

Approximate nutritional value for $^1/_{10}$ of recipe:

Calories: 20
Protein: 0.3 g
Carbohydrates: 4.2 g
Fat: Negl.
Fibre: 2.5 g

SEAFOOD SAUCE

Ingredients

5 tablespoons (100g) 'whole egg' mayonnaise (low-carbohydrate)
1 tablespoon light soy sauce
1 tablespoon light ketchup
1 teaspoon lemon juice

Method

Combine all ingredients and mix until well combined.

Approx. nutritional value per tablespoon

Calories: 97
Protein: 0.4 g
Carbohydrates: 1.6 g
Fat: 10 g
Fibre: 0 g

SMOKED SALMON HORS D'OEUVRES

Serves 4

Ingredients

150 g thinly sliced, smoked salmon
80 g light cottage cheese
few drops of Tabasco sauce (to taste)
1 tablespoon of light mayonnaise (low-carbohydrate)

Method

Cut salmon into strips, approximately 5 cm wide. Blend together remaining ingredients until smooth and well combined. Place the cheese mixture at one end of the salmon strips and roll, then secure with a toothpick. Serve as an appetiser or party finger-food.

Per serve:

Calories: 76
Protein: 13 g
Carbohydrates: 1.5 g
Fat: 2 g
Fibre: 0 g

SAVORY VOL-AU-VENT

Makes approx. 10

Ingredients

2 tablespoons of Parmesan cheese
1 egg
20 g/1 tablespoon of butter
50 g of almond meal
25 g of sesame seeds
Pinch of salt

Method

Preheat oven to 180/350 degrees.

Place all ingredients in a large mixing bowl and beat until well blended. Lightly brush a non-stick muffin tray with oil and press a thin layer of the mixture into each section. Bake for 12-15 minutes or until lightly browned. Allow to cool and fill with desired savory fillings.

Per vol-au-vent

Calories: 62.5
Protein: 2.1 g
Carbohydrates: negl.
Fat: 6 g
Fibre: 0.7 g

Used in conjunction with your newly acquired knowledge, these recipes can add a little creativity to your food preparation. Over the past ten years, I have worked on modifying my favorite recipes to create nutritious, yet tasty meals and treats. You need not deprive yourself of your favorite tastes. There is almost always a substitute or alternative which tastes just as good, if not better!

You will discover many lower-carbohydrate substitutes for almost every ingredient you encounter in a regular recipe. Some examples are:

Commonly used ingredients	Low-carbohydrate, nutritious substitutes
Plain flour	Soy flour/powder/Whey protein/ Soy protein/Almond meal
Mashed potato	Mashed vegetables, such as cauliflower
Thickening for sauces	Egg yolks/small amount of cornstarch
Bread crumbs	Almond meal/soy flour
Sugar	Splenda
Cooking oil	High oleic sunflower/safflower oils. [These are more stable to heat than other unrefined oils.] Butter/virgin olive oil
Commercial salad dressings	Balsamic vinegar, lemon juice, unrefined oils such as flaxseed and extra virgin olive oil

Protein powder

Whey protein is one of the best types of protein on the market due to the fact that it is easily absorbed by the body. Human mothers' milk is composed of 80% whey.

There are many to choose from in your healthfood shop and in some gymnasiums. Be sure to select one with no added sugars, for example, 'Aussie Bodies – Perfect Protein'.

Most of the ingredients used in the recipes are available from your local supermarket. Unrefined oils are available from the refrigerator of any reputable healthfood shop.

Low-fat, commercial products usually have a higher sugar/ carbohydrate content, to make up for the texture and taste lost in the reduction of fat. Be aware of this and read labels carefully! Many processed meats, salad dressings and condiments contain added starches and sugars. Even sugar-free products may still contain other forms of refined carbohydrates. It is a good idea to invest in a nutrition-counter booklet to ensure correct choices.

All the nutritional values of the recipes in this book have been calculated as accurately as possible. Due to variations in ingredients, some estimates may vary slightly.

How can I live without bread?

This seems to be the biggest obstacle for most people and it is probably due to the fact that bread is such a convenient food! It's easy to have a piece of toast in the morning or to grab a sandwich on the run. I find that most people who manage to resist the temptation for at least four weeks will survive and grow accustomed to life without it. It is not uncommon to look forward to tasting a slice of bread after a short break from it, only to find when you do, that it is not only disappointing, but also leaves you feeling bloated and nauseous.

There are so many foods on this eating plan that you have probably avoided for years thinking that they were fattening! If you really learn about, and get creative with all the 'new' foods that you can have, you will probably not even notice what you've left behind. And you will certainly notice the benefits!

ALL YOU NEVER WANTED TO KNOW ABOUT NUTRITION

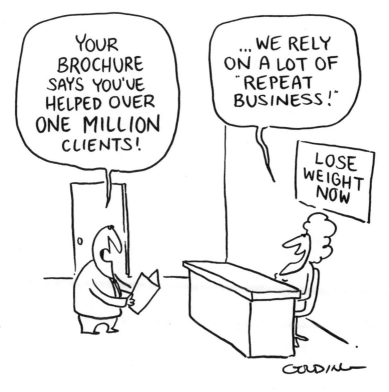

This section aims to give you some further information about:

- the major vitamins and minerals, where to find them, and why they are necessary
- carbohydrates, proteins, fats and antioxidants.

27
VITAMINS AND MINERALS

Vitamin A and Beta-carotene

Beta-carotene is the 'precursor' for vitamin A, which must undergo conversion to vitamin A within the body prior to absorption. Beta-carotene forms the pigment of the deep green and orange fruits and vegetables.

Functions

Vitamin A aids in the growth and repair of body tissues involving skin cells to help maintain soft, disease-free skin. Internally, it assists in protecting the mucous membranes of the nose, sinuses, lungs, eyelids, uterus, vagina, mouth, throat, stomach and intestines, thereby reducing susceptibility to infection. Vitamin A assists in the protection of the bladder and kidneys, as well as prompting the secretion of gastric juices necessary for protein digestion. Other functions include building strong bones and teeth, developing immunity and maintaining good eyesight.

Deficiencies

A lack of vitamin A may cause night blindness and other eye disorders, rough, dry skin, premature ageing, skin blemishes, loss of appetite, sties in the eyes, fatigue, weak immune system, bladder infections and brittle fingernails, just to name a few!

Sources

Carrots, liver, cod liver oil, butter, cheese, eggs, yellow/orange fruits and vegetables, e.g. spinach, capsicum, broccoli, tomato, rockmelon, avocado, peach, apricots, watermelon, pumpkin.

Vitamin B1 (Thiamine)

Functions

Vitamin B1 assists in starch, sugar and alcohol metabolism, stimulates appetite, keeps nerve cells healthy, and helps to maintain muscle tone in the stomach, intestines and the heart. Excessive consumption of sugar and/or alcohol will cause a depletion of vitamin B1.

Deficiencies

Symptoms of deficiency may include fatigue, loss of appetite, nightmares, lack of co-ordination, heart irregularities, low blood pressure, and a loss of mental alertness. Alcoholics are at the greatest risk of deficiency of vitamin B1.

Sources

Pork, organ meats, brewers yeast, bran and germ of wheat, nuts, egg yolks, sunflower seeds, chicken, meat and fish.

Vitamin B2 (Riboflavin)

Functions

Vitamin B2 is necessary for protein, carbohydrate and fat metabolism, as well as for growth and healthy skin. This vitamin is stored in the muscles and is used at times of physical exertion. Vitamin B2 also acts as an antioxidant, which tracks down abnormal cells in the body, such as those that cause cancer. Vitamin B2 is not stored for great lengths of time within the body, therefore it must be replenished regularly through the diet.

Deficiencies

Unlike vitamin B1, B2 is not found in a great variety of foods, therefore a deficiency can arise if the diet is unbalanced. Deficiencies in this vitamin manifest mainly in the skin and mucous membranes. The most common symptoms of B2 deficiency are cracks and sores in the corner of the mouth, lesions on the lips, a sore tongue, a feeling of grit inside the eyelids, burning of the eyes, dilation of the pupil, sensitivity to light, oily skin, eczema, or scaling around the nose, mouth and forehead. Some of the factors inhibiting absorption of vitamin B2 are heavy coffee and tea intake, bisulfite preservatives in foods, and use of diuretics or antacids. Commonly B2 and iron deficiencies occur at the same time.

Sources

Liver and other organ meats, pork, cheese, chicken, wheat germ, yoghurt, eggs, brewers yeast, almonds and fish.

Vitamin B3 (Nicotinic acid)

Functions

Vitamin B3 is an effective detoxificant, even for narcotics and alcohol. It is effective in improving circulation and reducing cholesterol levels in the blood. Vitamin B3 is vital to proper activity of the nervous system, health of the skin, tongue and tissues of the digestive system, and for the synthesis of sex hormones.

Deficiencies

There are many symptoms of B3 deficiency, including muscular weakness, fatigue, loss of appetite, indigestion, bad breath, ulcers, skin eruptions, insomnia, recurring headaches, tender gums and deep depression. Severe deficiencies can result in pellegra which is characterised by dermatitis, dementia, diarrhoea, rough, inflamed skin, tremors, nervous disorders and inflammation of the mucous membranes within the mouth and gastrointestinal tract.

Sources

Lean meats, poultry, tuna, salmon, swordfish, liver, pork, veal, peanuts, brewers yeast, wheat germ, desiccated liver tablets, avocado, sunflower seeds, mushrooms and eggs.

Vitamin B5 (Pantothenic acid)

Functions

Vitamin B5 stimulates the adrenal glands and increases production of cortisone and other adrenal hormones vital for healthy nerves and skin. B5 participates in the release of energy from protein, carbohydrates and fats, as well as being essential in the synthesis of cholesterol and fatty acids. Vitamin B5 can improve the body's ability to withstand stressful conditions and is important in the maintenance of a healthy digestive tract.

Deficiencies

Symptoms of deficiency may include abdominal pains, sensitivity to insulin, upper respiratory infections, skin disorders, low blood-sugar, duodenal ulcers and burning feet. The list of deficiency symptoms reflects impaired health of many tissues within the body and may arise due to lack of intestinal flora needed to synthesise this vitamin.

Sources

Organ meats, brewers yeast, egg yolks, and in yeasts, moulds, bacteria and individual cells of all animals and plants.

Vitamin B6 (Pyridoxine)

Functions

Vitamin B6 is required for the proper functioning of more than 60 enzymes and for normal amino acid synthesis. Vitamin B6 is essential in physical activity because it is involved in the release of glycogen from the liver and muscles. It plays a role in the multiplication of all cells and must be present for the production of blood cells and cells of the immune system. Vitamin B6 has been proven to assist in the correction of metabolic imbalances caused by oral contraceptives and may help alleviate a myriad of PMS symptoms.

Deficiencies

Vitamin B6 deficiencies may occur if a daily supply is not ingested. B6 is excreted in the urine and, within eight hours of ingestion, it is not found in the liver but is found exclusively in the muscles. The need for this vitamin is increased during pregnancy, lactation, exposure to radiation, ageing and the use of oral contraceptives. Symptoms of B6 deficiency may include anaemia, irritability, weakness, insomnia, skin problems, hair loss, low blood-sugar and low glucose tolerance, arthritis, an increase in urination, and water retention. In pregnancy, a B6 deficiency can lead to morning sickness, Carpal Tunnel Syndrome or still births. Estrogen therapy during menopause also depletes vitamin B6.

Sources

Meats, liver and other organ meats, tuna, prawns, salmon, egg yolks, nuts, avocado, carrots, wheat bran, sunflower seeds, many fresh vegetables and milk. Brewers yeast and desiccated liver are the best supplemental sources.

Vitamin B12

Functions

Vitamin B12 cannot be made synthetically and must be grown, like penicillin, in bacteria or moulds. It is necessary for normal metabolism of nerve tissue and is involved in protein, fat and carbohydrate metabolism. Vitamin B12 is essential for regeneration of red blood cells, maintenance of healthy nerves and mental abilities, in the production of DNA and haemoglobin, as well as assisting in the function of iron in the body. Vitamin B12 aids the body's absorption of Carotene or vitamin A conversion.

Deficiencies

A common reason for vitamin B12 deficiency is the lack of one or more gastric secretions necessary for its absorption. It is certainly not an uncommon deficiency. A lack of either B12 or Folic Acid will impair the development of rapidly growing blood cells in the bone marrow, producing anaemia of the large, red, blood cells. A deficiency is usually due to a problem with the absorption of the vitamin. This is known as 'the intrinsic factor'. Due to this intrinsic factor, deficiencies may be present even when a normal blood level exists. Symptoms of deficiency may include: pernicious anaemia, fatigue, pale skin, anorexia, weight loss, depression, weakness in the limbs, diminished reflex response and memory loss. Severe deficiency can lead to brain damage, where symptoms may include pins-and-needles, numbness, shooting pains, and hot and cold sensations. Alcohol can interfere with B12 absorption. B12 has been proven to improve the growth rate of children, help reduce the effects of bruising and has been successfully used to treat the symptoms of hangovers.

Sources

Organ and muscle meats, eggs, cheese, milk, milk products and fish. Animal proteins are the only significant source of natural B12 in substantial amounts.

Folic Acid (Folate)

Functions

Another one of the water-soluble B vitamin group, folic acid functions together with B12 and C in the breakdown of proteins. Folic acid is active in the role of cell division, and is a carrier in the formation of heme, the iron-containing protein in haemoglobin necessary for red blood-cell formation. It is necessary for normal brain function and is concentrated in the spinal fluid. It stimulates hydrochloric acid production to help prevent food poisoning and intestinal parasites. Folic acid aids the function of the liver, makes DNA duplication possible and may protect against colon cancer.

Deficiencies

Many factors can interfere with folic acid absorption and therefore it is quite a common deficiency. Antagonists include alcohol, illnesses involving vomiting or diarrhoea, smoking, stress, disease, oral contraceptives and estrogen. It is destroyed in foods exposed to high temperatures or light for long periods.

Deficiency is most common in alcoholics, pregnant women and the elderly. Deficiencies during pregnancy will increase the risk of Spina Bifida (spinal cord does not form properly) in the foetus. These days, supplements are usually recommended prior to and in the early stages of pregnancy. Because of the role it plays in the formation of red blood cells, a lack of folic acid can result in anaemia, which cannot be treated successfully with iron supplementation. Symptoms may include poor growth, greying hair, intestinal disturbances, metabolic disturbances, forgetfulness and mental sluggishness.

Sources

The word folate is derived from the term foliage, which indicates where this vitamin is found – in green, leafy vegetables such as broccoli, spinach, brussel sprouts and cabbage, as well as in oranges, beans, brewers yeast, liver green peas, avocado, wheat bran and almonds.

Vitamin C (Ascorbic acid)

Functions

Vitamin C is another water-soluble vitamin that strengthens the walls of the body cells and blood vessels, promotes healthy teeth, gums, bones and joints, and assists in the formation of collagen and connective tissue, the healing of wounds and burns, and the production of scar tissue. It aids iron absorption, stimulates the immune system and acts as an antioxidant to protect vitamins A, E and PUFAs from oxidation. Vitamin C's potency can be lost through exposure to light, heat and air. One of its primary functions is to maintain collagen, a protein necessary for the formation of connective tissue in the skin, ligaments and bones. Because vitamin C aids the formation of red blood cells it is active in prevention of haemorrhaging. There is strong support for vitamin C's protective effects against certain types of cancer. Large concentrations of the vitamin are found in the adrenal glands, which are active in times of stress. Humans, apes and guinea pigs are among the few species that need vitamin C in their food intake, as they are unable to synthesise the amount needed within the body. Vitamin C is eliminated from the body through urine and perspiration within 3–4 hours of consumption, therefore it must be supplied often throughout the day. Any excess of the vitamin carried through the bladder may prevent bladder cancer.

Deficiencies

Symptoms of vitamin C deficiency may include shortness of breath; rough, dry and scaly skin; impaired digestion; dry, split hair; broken blood-vessels; bleeding gums; bruising; nosebleeds; broken capillaries on the skin; swelling in the joints; anaemia; lowered immune resistance; and slow wound-healing.

Smoking is known to lower blood levels of vitamin C by up to 31%. Other antagonists include alcohol, pollution, some medications and cancer treatments, dialysis and many chronic illnesses.

Sources

The main sources of vitamin C are fresh fruit and vegetables, such as oranges, strawberries, broccoli, cabbage, kiwifruit, capsicum, grapefruit, cantaloupe, brussel sprouts, tomatoes.

Vitamin D

Functions

Vitamin D is a fat-soluble vitamin involved in the absorption and metabolism of calcium and phosphorus, and promotes their transport in and out of bones and teeth. The sun's ultraviolet rays activate a form of cholesterol in the skin and convert it into vitamin D. Most people receive sufficient sunlight to facilitate much of their vitamin D production, however, those who do not, may rely more on food intake or supplementation. This vitamin is necessary for the normal growth of teeth and bones in children. Without sufficient vitamin D, bones and teeth do not calcify properly. Vitamin D works best in the presence of vitamin A and is valuable in maintaining a stable nervous system, normal heart action and normal blood clotting.

Deficiencies

The symptoms of vitamin D deficiency are the same as those related to calcium deficiency. Rickets is an associated major disorder with symptoms being softening of the scull, bowing legs, spinal curvature, enlarged wrists, knees and ankle joints, poorly developed muscles, nervous irritability, muscle twitching and softening of the teeth. The cochlea, a bone in the middle ear, is thought to deteriorate without adequate vitamin D to facilitate calcium absorption. Alcohol, some medications and very little exposure to sunlight can increase the risk of vitamin D deficiency.

Sources

Fats and oils of fatty fish, for example sardines, herring, mackerel, tuna and salmon. Cod-liver oil, egg yolks, butter and cheese are also good sources of this vitamin.

Vitamin E (Tocopherol)

Functions

Vitamin E is another fat-soluble vitamin and is essential for all forms of oxygen-consuming life forms. Being an antioxidant, vitamin E opposes oxidation of substances within the body. It protects substances against oxidation by taking the brunt of the attack itself and sparing healthy cells. Fat oxidation results in the formation of free-radicals. These are highly destructive in the body if sufficient antioxidants are not present. Vitamin E makes it possible for cardiac and skeletal muscle to function with less oxygen requirement, therefore increasing endurance and stamina. Vitamin E is effective in preventing blood clots, dilating blood vessels, strengthening capillary walls and protecting red blood cells from poisons in the blood. This vitamin may be beneficial in reducing PMS symptoms, relieving cramps, enhancing immunity, preventing oxidation of LDL-cholesterol, and reducing the risk of heart disease and cancer.

Deficiencies

Some antagonists that inhibit absorption or destroy vitamin E are chlorine in drinking water, rancid fats and oils, the contraceptive pill, laxatives, estrogen, heat processing and frying, oxidation and ultra-violet light. The first sign of a deficiency is the rupture of red blood cells due to free-radical oxidation, making the cells fragile. Shrinkage of collagen (a connective tissue), muscle wasting, reduced adrenal and pituitary gland function, impaired iron absorption, and, in severe cases, damage to the liver and kidneys, are also related to deficiency in this vitamin. There is increasing evidence that vitamin E may be capable of slowing or even preventing Parkinson's Disease.

Sources

Cold-pressed oils, such as wheat-germ oil, safflower oil, sunflower and other seeds, almonds, hazelnuts and peanuts, soybean oil, tuna (canned in oil), peanut butter, wheat germ, avocado, spinach, olive oil, and egg yolks. Other sources are organ meats and desiccated liver.

Vitamin K

Functions

Vitamin K contributes to 4 of the 13 components necessary for blood-clot formation to prevent excessive bleeding. Vitamin K is fat-soluble and can be manufactured in the presence of bacteria in the intestinal tract. It plays a role in bone mineralisation and fracture healing, and may help to prevent osteoporosis. Rancid fats, radiation, x-rays, aspirin, industrial pollution, mineral oil in laxatives and excessive antibiotic use will destroy this vitamin. Unsaturated fatty acids and a low-carbohydrate diet increase the amounts produced by the intestinal flora.

Deficiencies

Those who follow a low-calorie diet or are on prolonged antibiotic therapy are at the greatest risk of deficiency in vitamin K. A deficiency may cause haemorrhages in any part of the body, including the brain, spinal cord, intestinal tract and nose. It may even cause miscarriage. Bruising or black and blue marks on the skin are another indication of vitamin K deficiency.

Sources

Some natural sources are kelp, alfalfa, green, leafy vegetables, cauliflower, cow's milk, yoghurt, egg yolks, safflower oil, fish-liver oils, liver and tomatoes.

Minerals

There are approximately 17 minerals, which have been found to be essential in human nutrition. Minerals also play a vital role in body growth and maintenance. All tissues and fluids within the body contain varying quantities of minerals. Included in these are bones, teeth, muscle, blood and nerve cells. Minerals are essential for strengthening skeletal structures, as well as maintaining the proper functions of the heart, brain, muscles and nervous system.

Minerals are not absorbed as easily as many vitamins within our body. They are utilised effectively when they become attached to amino acids (protein). For this reason, it is essential to consume complete proteins with each meal. If minerals do not attach to amino acids, they become bound by phytic acids (from cereals and grains) which prohibits their absorption.

The mineral balance within the body can be maintained in correct proportions by eating a wide variety of fresh, unrefined foods. This balance can be upset by certain diseases, extreme forms of dieting or during periods of physical or emotional stress. Minerals are not at as high a risk of destruction through cooking, as are vitamins, however, they are often lost in peeling or are poured down the drain in cooking water.

Minerals required in larger quantities are known as essential minerals. Those required in smaller quantities are referred to as trace minerals.

Aluminium

Aluminium is a trace mineral, but it can be dangerous or even fatal to the human body if consumed in excessive amounts. There is no apparent function of aluminium in human nutrition. This mineral may bind with other substances and vitamins in the system to prevent their absorption.

Aluminium can be found in tap water, table salt (to prevent caking), baking powder, foil and cookware utensils, and it can be used as a bleaching agent in flour and as an emulsifier in some cheeses.

Because there is no use for this mineral in the body, there are no deficiency effects or symptoms.

Boron

Boron is a trace mineral essential for healthy bones, as it assists in the absorption of calcium.

Boron is found in leafy vegetables, fruits and nuts. Any deficiencies in this mineral are rare if a variety of fresh, unprocessed foods is consumed.

Post-menopausal women have shown an increased production of active forms of estrogen and testosterone when supplementing with 3 milligrams of boron per day.

Cadmium

Cadmium is a toxic trace mineral found in refined foods, such as flour, rice and white sugar. 'Soft' water may leach cadmium from metal waterpipes.

Food refining processes disturb the balance of cadmium and zinc. If zinc levels are kept high, cadmium will be excreted, however, if zinc levels are depleted, the body will compensate with retention of a higher level of cadmium.

Because this is a toxic mineral, there are no symptoms of the effects of deficiencies in the body.

Calcium

With 99% of our calcium concentrated in our bones and teeth, and 1% in soft tissues, intracellular fluids and blood, it is the most abundant mineral in the body. The main function of calcium is to develop and maintain bone structure and rigidity. It is involved in the clotting process, nerve transmission, muscle stimulation, enzyme regulation, vitamin D metabolism and hormone functions, just to name a few of its uses. The calcium level of the bones is constantly fluctuating, dependent on the diet and the body's needs. Calcium is essential for easing insomnia and regulating heartbeat. When insufficient calcium is obtained from foods, the body leaches calcium from the bones. This loss over time may lead to osteoporosis (thinning of the bones). Calcium deficiencies are very common in human societies, with only one-third to one-half of the body's requirements being consumed. With the 'low-fat craze' sweeping the Western world, at the present time, many calcium-rich foods are being eliminated from the average diet.

The first signs of deficiency may be osteoporosis (fragile bones), or tetany, characterised by muscle cramps, numbness and tingling in the arms and legs. Other symptoms of calcium deficiency are rickets (causing bone malformation), hypertension, abnormal heart beat, cramps, joint pain, increased cholesterol, slow pulse rate, brittle nails, tooth decay and eczema.

Some of the factors that inhibit absorption and utilisation of calcium, or increase the need for more are excessive alcohol intake, smoking, pregnancy (higher levels used in the body), menopause, antacids, cortisone and a generally sedentary lifestyle.

Calcium is found in milk, yoghurt, cheese (with the exception of cottage), canned fish with edible bones (salmon and sardines), shellfish, almonds, broccoli, asparagus, cabbage and sesame seeds.

Chlorine (chloride)

This is another essential mineral. It helps to regulate the balance of acid and alkali in the blood, as well as acting as a stimulant for hydrochloric acid production (an enzymatic digestive juice in the stomach). Chlorine stimulates liver function, aids in joint and tendon maintenance and helps to distribute hormones.

Chlorine is provided in the diet through sodium chloride (table salt), and is found in kelp, ripe olives, seafood and meats.

Chlorine is sometimes added to tap water to destroy water-born diseases such as typhoid and hepatitis.

A deficiency of this mineral can cause hair and tooth loss, poor muscle contraction and impaired digestion. Losses of chlorine usually indicate a loss of sodium.

Chromium

Chromium is an essential mineral, which is now recognised as an important component in carbohydrate metabolism. It stimulates the activity of enzymes involved in the metabolism of glucose for energy and the synthesis of fatty acids and cholesterol. Chromium increases the effectiveness of insulin, therefore helping to prevent hypoglycaemia (low blood sugar) and diabetes.

The best sources of chromium are brewer's yeast, liver, beef, lamb, meats and cheeses, mushrooms and black pepper.

The refining of foods is a probable cause of chromium loss in our foods, as well as a high intake of sugars and other refined carbohydrates. Strenuous exercise, pregnancy (due to the large amounts the foetus uses) and viral infections can lead to a deficiency in chromium.

Cobalt

Cobalt is an essential mineral and an integral part of vitamin B12. It is necessary for normal functioning and maintenance of red blood cells. Cobalt cannot be synthesised within the body and so we must depend on animal sources for sufficient supply. Vegetarians are more susceptible to deficiencies than are meat eaters.

The best sources of cobalt are meat, organ meats, cabbage, spinach, lettuce, seafood, nuts and milk. A deficiency of cobalt may result in pernicious anaemia.

Copper

Copper is a trace mineral found in every tissue of the body. During periods of growth, copper is concentrated in the developing tissues. It is involved in the processes of respiration, the production of collagen, the prevention of rancidity of PUFAs and it helps cell membranes stay healthy. Copper is essential in the formation of myelin sheaths (protective covers) around nerve fibres, and is necessary for proper bone formation.

Some of the best sources of copper are liver, almonds, brazil nuts, peanuts, green, leafy vegetables, shellfish, crustaceans, kidneys, cauliflower, avocados, organ meats, wheat germ, eggs and poultry.

Symptoms of deficiency may include general weakness, impaired respiration, ineffective use of iron and protein, diarrhoea and stunted growth. People who consume excessive fructose (fruit sugar) or antacids are at higher risk of copper losses.

Fluorine (Fluorides)

Although fluoride is present in soil, water, plants and all animal tissue, it has not been acknowledged as an essential mineral in humans. Research on fluoride shows that it helps reduce the formation of acid in the mouth due to carbohydrate ingestion, therefore reducing the risk of tooth decay. Traces of this mineral have beneficial effects within the body, however, excessive amounts are definitely harmful. Fluoride may inhibit or even destroy other vitamins and enzymes, and appears to be especially antagonistic toward brain tissues.

Sources of fluoride include drinking water, fish and seafood, milk, cheese, meat and tea. Fluoride levels in plant foods vary greatly depending on the amount of the mineral in the soil and the fertilisers and sprays used.

Although unusual, deficiencies may lead to tooth decay and poor tooth development.

Iodine (iodide)

Iodine is a trace mineral which is converted to iodide in the body. It plays an important role in the development and functioning of the thyroid gland and the hormones it secretes. Iodine assists in the regulation of the body's production of energy, promotes growth and development, stimulates the metabolism, and promotes the health of hair, nails and teeth.

Plant and animal sealife absorb this mineral from seawater and are good sources of iodine.

White, deep-water fish, brown seaweed, kelp, garlic, sesame seeds and spinach contain among the highest quantities of iodine. Mushrooms can be a good source if grown in iodine-rich soil.

A deficiency can result in goiter (enlarged thyroid), hypothyroidism (low production of thyroid hormone), hardening of the arteries, obesity, slow metabolic rate, dry hair, rapid pulse, nervousness and irritability. Some raw foods, if consumed in excessive amounts, can interfere with iodine absorption, such as cabbage and nuts.

Iron

Iron combines with protein to form haemoglobin (the red-pigment which carries oxygen in the blood). This mineral is concentrated in every living cell of the body. Haemoglobin transports oxygen in the blood from the lungs to the tissues, which need oxygen to maintain basic life functions. Because the quality of the blood is improved by the presence of iron, this increases the resistance to stress and disease, and improves energy production, growth in children and oxygen transportation throughout the body.

The best sources of iron are liver, desiccated liver, eggs, oysters and most organ meats. Other less potent sources are leafy, green vegetables, peas, chicken, strawberries, pumpkin and salmon. The iron found in animal protein is more readily absorbed than that found in vegetables.

Pregnancy, menstruation and blood loss due to injury will deplete stores of iron. Alcohol, antacids and excessive consumption of tea and coffee reduce the absorption of iron. Consuming foods high in vitamin C, in conjunction with those rich in iron, will enhance absorption.

The most common symptom of iron deficiency is anaemia, characterised by a reduction in haemoglobin in the red blood cells. Twenty-eight milligrams of iron is lost monthly by menstruating women. Some symptoms of anaemia are constipation, lustreless hair, brittle nails, nail ridges, shortness of breath, lethargy, headache, pale skin, and an impaired immune response.

Magnesium

Magnesium is an essential mineral, with 70% of the body's supply located in the bones and 30% in cellular fluids and some soft tissue. Magnesium is essential for the health of the heart, muscles and nervous system. It assists calcium in the maintenance of strong bones and is essential for muscle contraction and proper nerve function. A magnesium-rich diet may reduce the risk of asthma attacks due to its ability to relax the lining of the breathing passages and lungs.

Magnesium is widely distributed in foods, such as green vegetables, seafood, nuts (brazil, almonds, cashews and peanuts), avocado, apples, apricots, wheat bran, salmon, tuna, meat and yoghurt.

Deficiencies are not uncommon, as magnesium can be refined out of many foods during processing. Deficiencies are more likely to occur in diabetics, the elderly, when there is chronic diarrhoea or vomiting, when consuming high levels of zinc, fluoride or vitamin D, and where diets are high in carbohydrate and low in calories. Symptoms may include irregular heart rhythm, lack of co-ordination, muscle twitches, weakness and depression.

Manganese

Manganese is a trace mineral that acts in the body as an antioxidant. Manganese also plays a role in activating many enzymes necessary for utilisation of other vitamins and minerals. It is a catalyst in the synthesis of fatty acids and cholesterol, as well as assisting in regulation of blood-sugar levels.

Avocados, seaweed, egg yolks, nuts, seeds, blueberries, pineapples, spinach, and green vegetables are good sources of manganese. The content of manganese in vegetables will vary due to the mineral content of the soil. A large portion of manganese is lost in the processing of many foods.

A deficiency in this mineral can lead to the inability to remove excess sugar from the blood, causing diabetes. Dizziness, ear noises and loss of hearing can occur in adults. Seizures may be triggered in epileptics in the case of a manganese deficiency.

Phosphorus

This is the second-most abundant mineral found in the body. Phosphorus plays an important role in almost every chemical reaction in the body. It stimulates muscle contractions, including the heart muscle and it is important in the utilisation of protein, carbohydrates and fats for growth, maintenance and repair within the body. The B vitamins and many enzymes need phosphorus to become active.

Protein-rich foods are good sources of phosphorus, for example milk and dairy products, meat, fish, poultry and eggs, as well as asparagus, garlic, seeds and nuts.

A deficiency in this mineral may cause lack of appetite, weight loss or obesity, irregular breathing, mental and physical fatigue, and nervous disorders. Those at risk are diabetics, alcoholics, those with malabsorption problems and those using excessive amounts of antacids.

Potassium

This is an essential mineral, with 98% found in the intracellular fluid of the body. Potassium and sodium together help to regulate water balance in the body. Potassium also regulates the transfer of nutrients to the cells of the body and is essential in muscle contraction, beating of the heart, energy production and protein synthesis. A deficiency is most common in people on diuretic drugs, or in cases of vomiting and diarrhoea, high salt, coffee or tea intake, extensive physical exertion (therefore perspiration), an inadequate intake of fruits and vegetables, or excessive refined sugar intake. Symptoms may include muscular weakness, confusion, irregular heartbeat, and poor reflexes.

Potassium is found in all animal and plant cells. Some good food sources are apples, avocado, apricots, cantaloupe, oranges, peaches, nuts, sunflower seeds, green beans, cabbage, spinach, pumpkin, tomatoes, meat, chicken, fish, eggs, milk and yoghurt.

Selenium

Selenium is considered an essential nutrient and is found in small quantities throughout the body. Selenium can be used by the body as a preventative substance against many diseases, including cancer, stroke, arteriosclerosis, arthritis and emphysema. Selenium is an antioxidant and appears to preserve elasticity of the tissue. All age-associated diseases are affected by the functions of selenium. The selenium content of food depends on the levels of the mineral in the environment they are derived from. Selenium works closely with vitamin E in the production of antibodies, binding of toxic minerals and the promotion of normal growth and fertility. It assists in the maintenance of cells, including those of the heart, by ensuring adequate oxygen is supplied.

Good food sources of selenium are brewer's yeast, organ and muscle meats, fish and shellfish, brazil and cashew nuts, sesame and sunflower seeds, broccoli, cabbage, cucumber, garlic, eggs and dairy products.

A deficiency in this mineral may lead to premature ageing, diminished vision, cataracts, growth retardation, muscular dystrophy and certain forms of cancer. Some recent Australian studies show that a selenium deficiency may relate to Sudden Infant Death Syndrome (SIDS).

Silicon

This is the most abundant mineral and is found in the tissues of the skin, fingernails, bones, lungs, trachea, lymph nodes, tendons and aorta. It is not recognised as an essential mineral in humans, however, it is necessary for the integrity of connective tissues in the body, such as tendons, cartilage and collagen. It works with calcium to make our bones strong and prevent osteoporosis. Silicon is known to act against toxic minerals in the body, including aluminium, which may protect the body against Alzheimer's Disease.

The best sources of silicon are hard drinking water, plant fibre, seafood, capsicum, green, leafy vegetables or in supplement form.

Sodium

Sodium is an essential mineral. Approximately half of our sodium is found in the extracellular fluids of the body, whilst the other 50% is found in the bones. Along with potassium, sodium helps to regulate fluid and the acid/alkali balance within the body. Sodium and potassium are also involved in muscle contraction and nerve stimulation. Sodium prevents the build up of other minerals in the bloodstream, is involved in oxygen transportation and aids digestion. Sodium can be found in many food sources, the most common being table salt.

Plant sources have less sodium than animal sources. Highly processed foods may contain an excessive quantity of sodium, therefore creating a mineral imbalance if consumed in large quantities.

Some natural sources of sodium are table salt, seafood, kelp, celery, milk, poultry and meat. Other forms of sodium are present in soy sauce, MSG, nitrate, nitrite, baking soda, baking powder, and other spices, condiments and additives.

Deficiencies are uncommon, however, they may occur in cases of vomiting, diarrhoea, extreme perspiration, or any large, fluid losses. Symptoms of deficiency may include intestinal gas, weight loss, inability to concentrate, low blood sugar, heart palpitations, and muscle weakness.

Zinc

Zinc is an essential trace mineral, occurring in the body in larger quantities than other trace minerals. Zinc plays an important role in the maintenance of a strong immune system, as well as improving the healing of wounds. Zinc promotes normal absorption of the B vitamins, regulates testosterone in the prostate, and is an important constituent in many of the body's enzymes.

Zinc concentrations in our food can be diminished due to poor soil quality and in processing. By consuming natural, unprocessed foods such as wheat germ, brewer's yeast, pumpkin and sunflower seeds, nuts and high levels of protein, zinc levels should remain at an adequate level within the body. Other protein sources include oysters, beef, organ meats, eggs, turkey, lamb, scallops, lobster and pork.

Two factors responsible for deficiencies in this mineral are an unbalanced diet (high in grains and low in animal protein) and consumption of alcohol. Athletes, vegetarians and dieters may be deficient in zinc. Symptoms of deficiency include poor appetite, loss of taste or smell, slow wound healing, susceptibility to infections, excessive hair loss, reduced sexual libido, stretch-marks on the skin, white-spots on the nails and irregular menstrual cycles.

28
PROTEINS

Proteins are any of a large group of nitrogenous compounds of high molecular weight that are essential constituents of all living organisms. They consist of one or more chains of amino acids (organic compounds that are the component molecules of proteins).

Proteins provide the building materials for the basic cell structure of our heart, brain, blood, nails, hair, internal organs and skin – in fact, for every living cell in our body.

Apart from water, protein is more plentiful than any other substance in the body. Constituting approximately 12% of our total weight, it is responsible for growth and development within the body. Our bones, nerves and other body tissues are composed of mostly protein. Collagen, an important protein, forms the protein base of teeth, skin elasticity, the material for tendons and ligaments, and the strength in the arterial walls, and it assists in the production of scar-tissue formation. If there is an absence of 'energy' foods (carbohydrate and fat), protein can be used as a source of heat and energy for the body at a rate of 4 calories per gram.

Protein also performs the following functions:
- It controls the pH (acid/alkaline) level of blood and tissues.
- With the aid of some minerals, it helps regulate the body's water balance.
- Protein in the form of enzymes helps fight bacteria, infection and disease.
- Protein is responsible for the production of milk in lactating mothers.
- It performs an important role in blood clotting.
- 'Transport proteins' are responsible for picking up nutrients and moving them in and out of the cells. They move fat, fat-soluble vitamins, water-soluble vitamins and minerals to every cell in the body.

- The protein, 'haemoglobin', carries oxygen from the lungs to the cells of organs.

The digestion time of protein foods is usually around 3–5 hours. During digestion, protein is broken down into usable particles. These are the amino acids. There are 22 amino acids in a complete protein. All but nine of these can be produced by the body, therefore, 13 amino acids are known as 'non-essential' and 9 as 'essential' because they must be supplied by the diet. Some non-essential amino acids can become essential in the event of stress. The body loses protein in situations of physical and emotional stress, such as surgery, emotional trauma, illness/disease or wounds. This creates extra demand on the body to consume more protein in the diet to rebuild or replace tissues that no longer function effectively. To enable the body to utilise protein properly, all amino acids must be present at the same time. If just one amino acid is missing, protein synthesis can cease altogether and all amino acids will be reduced to the proportion of the low or missing amino.

When a food contains all 22 amino acids, it is referred to as a 'complete' protein. If a food is low in, or missing one amino acid, it is referred to as an 'incomplete' protein. As a general rule, animal proteins are 'complete' proteins, while most vegetable sources are 'incomplete'. The only method of receiving a complete protein from incomplete sources, is to combine them correctly in order to balance the content of amino acids. Soy protein is one of the only plant-derived proteins considered a complete source.

Two diseases may develop due to a protein deficiency. They are Kwashiorkor and Marasmus Disease.

Kwashiorkor results from a severe protein deficiency and usually affects just-weaned children and those who are going through rapid growth phases. The body becomes swollen with fluid and a fatty liver develops.

Marasmus is basically due to starvation. A lack of protein and calories in general is involved. This disease is found in overpopulated, poor areas and where infant formulas are not adequate. In adults, protein deficiency can manifest in symptoms such as depression, lack of stamina, weakness, poor resistance to infection, and impaired healing of wounds and general recovery from disease.

The minimum daily requirement of protein for an adult is 1 gram of complete protein per kilogram of body weight. As with most recommended-daily-intake (RDI's) amounts, this is the minimum, not necessarily the optimum amount of protein that can maintain growth and good health in the average person. If we take into account factors like pollution, pregnancy, lactation, rapid growth phases, stress, smoking, exercise, illness, medication, etc. then this RDI is probably nowhere near your requirement.

Current Australian Recommended Daily Intake of protein per kilogram of body weight:

Infants

0-6 months	2 grams/kilo
6–12 months	1.6 grams/kilo

Children

1-3 years	1.2 grams/kilo
4-7 years	1 gram/kilo
8-11 years	1 gram/kilo

Males

12-15 years	1 gram/kilo
16-18 years	1 gram/kilo
19 years +	.75 gram/kilo

Females

12-15 years	1 gram/kilo
16-18 years	1 gram/kilo
19 years +	.75 gram/kilo

29
CARBOHYDRATES

Carbohydrates are any of a large group of organic compounds, including sugars, such as sucrose, and polysaccharides, such as cellulose, glycogen and starch, that contain carbon, hydrogen and oxygen. All sugars and starches are carbohydrates. Carbohydrates are divided into two categories.

'Simple' carbohydrates: single sugars composed of one molecule and requiring only 30 minutes or less for digestion. Simple carbohydrates are glucose, as well as fructose (fruit sugar) and lactose (milk sugar), which the liver converts into glucose.

'Complex' carbohydrates: starch and glycogen are composed of many different chains of glucose. They require a longer time for enzymes to break down their parts into simple sugars and then glucose for absorption (approximately 2–3 hours digestion time).

Some of the glucose is used as fuel by the body, while the rest is converted into glycogen and is stored in the liver and muscles. Any excess is converted to triglycerides and accumulates under the skin and throughout the body as fat reserves. When the body burns stored-fat reserves, it breaks triglycerides back down to the form of glucose, and weight loss results.

When carbohydrate foods that are lacking in essential nutrients are consumed (processed foods), they are often referred to as 'empty calories'. Overindulgence in these foods can result in simultaneous malnourishment and obesity. Many carbohydrate foods can cause an immediate rise in blood-sugar levels. To correct this, the body will automatically release insulin, which is designed to bring blood sugar back to a normal level. Unfortunately, simple sugars trigger such an extreme rise in blood sugar, that insulin tends to over-compensate and the blood sugar is returned to a level lower than the starting point. When this level drops, you may experience a demand by the body to stabilise blood sugar to a normal level again and this causes a craving for more sweet foods and, possibly, dizziness, fatigue, nervousness and headache. Excess consumption of these refined foods can also create a B vitamin deficiency.

A modest amount of unrefined carbohydrate foods must be part of a balanced and healthy diet. To gain maximum nutritional benefits, the diet should comprise mainly fibrous vegetables, nuts, seeds, small quantities of unrefined grains and fruit, to provide fibre and nourishment.

To date, there is no documented research which shows that the requirement of carbohydrates recommended by most dietitians (60% of total calories) is essential for optimum health, however, there is evidence that shows that an over-consumption leads to numerous health problems, including diabetes and obesity. As demonstrated by diabeties, high blood-glucose levels have been proven to be extremely detrimental to our health, causing many degenerative disorders and accelerating tissue ageing. These disorders arise in diabetics due to their inability to control blood-sugar levels with efficient insulin response, therefore blood-sugar levels remain much higher than in the average person. This in turn fuels a process known as 'glycation', where sugars (glucose and others, such as fructose) react spontaneously with proteins within the body such as collagen (skin protein), blood vessels, myelin (nerve protective sheaths) and connective tissues. This reaction forms 'cross-linked', sugar-damaged protein. Cross-linking is a process that stiffens tissue, resulting in aged skin, hardening of the arteries and many other degenerative symptoms. The degree of damage is proportional to the sugar concentration in the system. This process does occur in the non-diabetic person who has a higher than necessary intake of simple sugars and carbohydrate foods, which cause high-glucose levels. Controlling our blood-sugar levels throughout our lives should contribute to 'young-for-the-age' tissue structure.

Apart from vegetables, fruit, nuts and seeds, most other sources of starch and carbohydrates have been processed in some way.

The processing of food was invented to 'feed the masses'...cheaply! Bread, pasta, cereal, sugar....it's all processed and it's all cheap.

Manufacturers encourage the consumption of processed foods by extolling the benefits to our health! By the time most of these products have been prepared, there is little, if any, of the natural food's nutritional attributes remaining. Husks, and therefore fibre have been removed and discarded, and natural oils containing anti-oxidant vitamins have been destroyed by exposure to heat, light and oxygen. The cardboard boxes that are used for packaging would probably be more nutritious!

Man cannot live on bread alone!

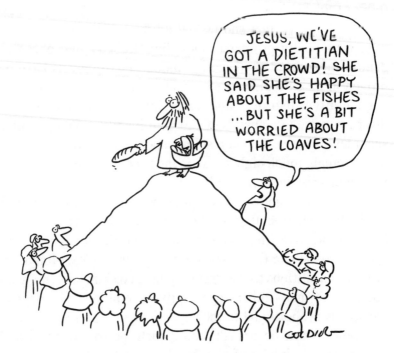

> JESUS, WE'VE GOT A DIETITIAN IN THE CROWD! SHE SAID SHE'S HAPPY ABOUT THE FISHES ...BUT SHE'S A BIT WORRIED ABOUT THE LOAVES!

The following table represents the nutritional profile of some widely consumed carbohydrate foods, including their National recommended daily intake (RDI).

Judging by this table, if one were to consume these refined foods as a staple dietary source, it would be necessary to consume around 30 slices of bread, or 15 cups of rice to achieve the bare minimum nutritional requirement, daily. (Equivalent to 2070 calories in bread, or 3075 calories in rice!)

Carbohydrates can be manufactured in the body from some amino acids and the glycerol component of fats, therefore the U.S. National Research Council lists no specific requirement (RDI) for the consumption of these foods as a primary energy source.

Nutritional profile of bread and rice

Nutrient	Bread – whole wheat, 1 slice		Rice – white long grain: $\frac{1}{2}$ cup	
	Amount	% RDI	Amount	% RDI
Calories	69 cals	3	102 cals	4.5
Protein	2.7 g	3	2.1 g	2.5
Carbohydrates	12.9 g	4	23 g	7
Fat	1.2 g	2	.23 g	0
Cholesterol	–	–	–	–
Saturated Fat	0.258	2	0.5 g	.5
Sodium	148.0 mg	6	0.5 mg	0
Dietary Fibre	0 g	0	0 g	0
Calcium	20 mg	2	8 mg	1
Iron	0.93 mg	6	.8 g	6
Vitamin A	–	–	–	–
Beta–carotene	–	–	–	–
Vitamin E	–	–	–	–
Thiamin B1	0.79 mg	7	.12 mg	11
Riboflavin B2	0.052 mg	3	.01 mg	.5
NiacinB3	0.970 mg	6	1.15 mg	7
Cobalamin B12	–	–	–	–
Vitamin C	–	–	–	–

30
FAT

Fat is any of a class of naturally occurring soft, greasy solids that are present in some plants and in the adipose tissue of animals forming a reserve energy source.

Fat is essential in the diet to facilitate transport and absorption of fat-soluble vitamins, A, D, E and K, many of which have an anti-oxidant effect on the body, protecting us from cancer and keeping our immune system strong. Seldom are we reminded of the benefits of certain fats in the diet and their necessary role in maintaining good health. Without fat in our diet, we tend to consume more calories due to unsatisfied hunger pangs. Fats, due to slower digestive absorption (approximately 5–8 hours), will help to sustain our blood sugar at a more consistent level. Fat is involved in the manufacturing process of our sex and adrenal hormones, the maintenance of body temperature, shielding nerves, organs and muscles, converting sun to vitamin D from cholesterol and it should contribute around 30% of our total calories. In the pursuit of good health, much of the population is aiming to keep their total fat intake below 30% of their total calories. It is not the quantity, but the quality of the fats and oils we are consuming that predict our state of wellbeing.

Fats are the most concentrated form of energy in the body, yielding 9 calories per gram. The substances that give fats their different flavors, textures and melting points are called fatty acids. These fatty acids are the building blocks of fats, much like amino acids are the building blocks of protein.

Unsaturated fatty acids (UFAs), found in most fish and plant sources, have points in chemical attachment that are missing. When only one point is missing, they are known as monounsaturated fatty acids (MFA). When two points are missing they are known as polyunsaturated fatty acids (PUFA). UFAs are usually liquid at room temperature. Some of their most common sources are vegetable oils, nuts, seeds, corn, safflower, sunflower and olives.

Saturated fatty acids (SFAs) are usually solid at room temperature, and, with the exception of palm and coconut oil are derived from animal sources – meats, milk, eggs, cheese, etc.

The modern diet is composed of too much processed animal and vegetable fats and not enough essential fats in their natural state.

The average consumption of essential fatty acids has fallen to only 20% of that consumed in diets 100 years ago. There has been a concerted effort over this century to remove Omega 3 fats from commercial foods as it does spoil and become rancid quite easily, inhibiting the manufacturers' desired shelf-life. Approximately 80% of our fat intake is derived from vegetable oils, primarily PUFAs.

Of all fatty acids in existence, the body can manufacture all it needs from available protein, carbohydrates and fats in the diet, with the exception of three essential groups:

- Linoleic Acid (LA or Omega 6)
- Alpha –Linolenic Acids (LNA or Omega 3)
- Gamma – Linolenic Acid (GL A).

They are known as essential fatty acids (EFAs) because they must be supplied through the diet. They are necessary for healthy blood and arteries, nerves and normal growth.

EFA's assist in regulating cholesterol metabolism and maintaining and regulating the functions and integrity of all cell membranes (being composed primarily of fat). They serve as precursors to prostaglandins (PGs), crucial components involved in the regulation of nearly every bodily function.

The more saturated fats you consume (from sources such as animal products), the higher the requirement for EFAs to create a balance.

A deficiency in EFAs can lead to a reduction in the number and size of brain cells, as well as a lack of communication between cells, leading to impaired learning, growing and thinking abilities.

Omega 3 is derived from cold water ocean fish, flaxseed oil (50%), hemp oil (20%), canola oil (10%), soy bean oil (5–7%), green, leafy vegetables (spinach), sea vegetables and pumpkin seeds. Sources of Omega 3 are primarily derived from colder climates. It is active in the maintenance of visual function, youthful skin texture, blood clotting, and prevention of cancer, heart disease and hypertension. A diet high in fish oil may help to alleviate arthritis, lupus, migraine, cancers of the colon, breast, prostate and pancreas, and it prevents excess calcium excretion. The ratio between Omega 6 and Omega 3 must be balanced. The American Health Foundation, New York, reported a study in cancer research that used corn oil due to its richness in Omega 6 fatty acids and fish oil for its Omega 3 properties. The findings confirmed that corn oil alone (without an Omega 3 balancing ratio) increased the multiplicity of colon carcinomas. The fish oil (Omega 3) produced the opposite effect due to efficient prostaglandin synthesis. Deep-water fish, such as herring, salmon, mackerel, bluefish and sardines are highest in essential oils.

A deficiency in Omega 3 is not uncommon, often showing symptoms including eczema, psoriasis, dry skin, brittle nails, tingling sensations in the arms and legs, high blood pressure, high triglycerides, fluid retention and immune dysfunction.

Omega 6 is derived from seeds of plants and is in oils produced from the seeds, primarily from warm climates. These include safflower oil (80%), sunflower oil, evening primrose oil (72%), borage oil (34%), corn oil, sesame oil, flaxseed oil (20%) and hemp oil (50%). These fatty acids are important for the transport and breakdown of cholesterol. Balance of the Omega 3 and 6 fatty acids is essential, otherwise, as with many nutrients, a deficiency may be created if only one is consumed. The ideal ratio between the two is Omega 6 (3 parts) to Omega 3 (1 part). This can be achieved quite simply through our food choices, or by adding the oil to our daily diet. They are very mild tasting oils and can be added to salad dressings or any other foods. (Approx. requirement of the average adult is 2 tablespoons of combined 3 and 6 oil daily.) An Omega 6 deficiency can produce eczema, skin eruptions, hair loss, excessive perspiration/thirst, failure of wound healing, arthritis and infection susceptibility.

It is important that these oils are kept in the refrigerator at all times and are never heated or used for cooking purposes. You can buy specific 'high oleic' safflower oil which is an extra-stable product ideal for cooking. Butter and olive oil are also quite stable to heat. Essential fatty acids will become damaged (trans-fatty acids) if used for cooking.

Both Omega 3 and Omega 6 form the membranes (outer protective lining) of billions of cells within the body. They control the way cholesterol works in our system and compose large parts of the brains active tissue. These essential fats become prostaglandins, playing key roles in regulating the cardiovascular, immune, digestive and reproductive systems.

GLA is found in borage oil (20%+), blackcurrant seed oil (15%+) and evening primrose oil (9%).

Human milk is very high in GLA, which may explain the superior health of breastfed infants as opposed to those fed with GLA deficient formulas. GLA has been shown to have the following benefits:

- reducing body fat
- lowering cholesterol
- reducing blood pressure
- healing eczema
- relieving rheumatoid arthritis
- slowing the progression of multiple sclerosis
- relieving menstrual pain
- improving acne in combination with zinc
- improving behaviour of hyperactive children
- improving fingernails
- alleviating hangovers
- improving calcium absorption from the GI tract
- increasing efficiency of brown fat utilisation.

Deficiencies may cause:

- hair loss
- swollen joints
- dry skin
- irritability
- lethargy
- infection

- infertility
- poor liver function
- poor tissue structure.

It may take as long as 6–8 weeks to show the benefits of additional dietary GLA.

Oleic acid (Omega 9) is found in olives (75%), almonds, avocados, peanuts, pecans, cashews, macadamias, land animals and butter. They are not essential fats because they can be produced by the body, however, they are considered a healthy addition to the diet.

Prostaglandins (PGs) are fatty acids with hormone-like functions which regulate all cell activity. There are over 30 PGs known today and they are made from Omega 3 and 6 fatty acids.

Functions of PGs (known as P1 and 3) include:

- reducing cell division in malignant tissue (retarding cancer growth)
- stopping blood platelets from sticking together (reducing risk of heart disease/stroke)
- promoting production of normal T-cells (enhancing immune system)
- preventing arthritis and auto-immune diseases (in animal studies)
- promoting healing and repair
- enhancing thermostat and calorie-loss mechanisms within the body
- enhancing efficiency of digestive and reproductive systems.

Prostaglandins are not stored by the body, therefore must be manufactured on site when needed for regulatory tasks. This can only occur if adequate fatty acids are immediately available. These PGs influence the processes of many important functions, including blood pressure, blood clotting, blood-sugar levels, menstrual cramping, gastrointestinal secretions, fertility, reproduction, immunity, inflammation and pain. Disorders such as arthritis, asthma, migraine, glaucoma, diabetes and cancer can be a result of an undesirable PG balance.

Aspirin is often used as a 'blood-thinning' agent which enhances prostaglandins' ability to do their work.

The human body uses essential fatty acids (EFAs) for structural and metabolic functions, as opposed to a primary energy source. This indicates that these fats are far less likely to create an increase in body-fat levels.

On the contrary, EFAs have actually been shown to assist the body in burning fat more efficiently.

Ugly fats

Margarine and vegetable shortening have been through a process known as partial-hydrogenation to solidify these unsaturated fatty acids. This process allows manufacturers to transform 'cheap' oils into semi-liquid or other textures, which are spreadable and have a long shelf-life. These are known as trans-fatty acids (TFAs). Partially-hydrogenated vegetable fats are commonly found at a level of 30-53% of the fats in commercial food products. Margarine, shortening, french fries, sweets, bakery products and salad oils are just a few of our daily food items containing TFAs. These are now commonly known to be quite dangerous to our health, being linked to impaired EFA absorption, degeneration of the protective cell membranes (lining), and causing allergy and decreased immunity, as well as the formation of cancer.

These fats have been distorted to a state where enzymes can no longer recognise them – rendering us incapable of digesting them. This means that they are treated as foreign substances by our body.

This can be compared with changing the lock, therefore the key no longer fits. These trans-fatty acids are known to produce alterations in adipose (fat) cell size and number. The quantity of trans-fatty acids in our diet is increasing rapidly, yet there is little data available on the rate of consumption, to date.

The 60 grams of margarine/shortening consumed each day in the average diet contains twice as many 'toxic food additives' as are found in the 2,640 grams of total food consumed by the average man (1,740 grams by women) each day.

Totally hydrogenated oils are 'dead'. They have no Omega 3 and 6, no UFAs, TFAs or saturated fatty acids. Because they are dead, they do not spoil, therefore maintaining a long shelf-life and exposure to heat. Obviously perfect for manufacturers. These oils do, however, contain altered fat molecules and traces of chemicals (namely nickel and aluminium), which are toxic. There is now strong evidence showing a link between aluminium and the development of Alzheimer's Disease. These fats are often used in products such as chocolate.

Most people would be amazed if they were aware of some of the foods containing processed oils and fats. 'Brominated oils' are made from highly processed olive, cottonseed, corn, sesame and soybean oils. These oils are commonly used in commercially packaged fruit juice to prevent 'rings' of residue around bottlenecks. These oils have been banned in Holland and Germany.

Deep frying

During the process of frying with unstable oils, vitamin E and Beta-carotene are destroyed and the production of free radicals and trans-fatty acids begins. Generally, frying temperatures required for cooking food are far too high. If a food begins to brown, it has been burned ... therefore fats have been damaged.

Burned proteins become carcinogenic (cancer causing) acrolein, starches and sugars are browned through molecular destruction and smoke is created by destruction of fatty acids and glycerol. The most unsuitable oils for frying are those high in EFAs (unrefined). The fats least damaged during the frying process include butter, peanut oil, sesame oil, canola oil, olive oil (low-temp) or 'high-oleic' safflower oil/sunflower oils.

Trans-fatty acids ... Butter or margarine?

It was not until 1963 that polyunsaturated margarine was introduced in Australia.

Table margarine made from animal fat was still a component of the food supply in 1983, but had virtually disappeared by 1985. By 1992 polyunsaturated margarine made up 73% of the total margarine market. The consumption of butter has decreased steadily since the early 1950s, with table margarine becoming the second-largest contributor to the fat supply in our daily diet, along side cooking oils.

To process a vegetable oil (UFA) as in the manufacturing of margarine, butter substitutes and vegetable shortenings, the oil must be partially hydrogenated. This requires an operation which forces hydrogen into the oil molecules under high temperature and pressure, artificially saturating it, rendering the product solid at room temperature, therefore resembling butter.

Although we purchase these products for their convenience – they remain solid, yet soft and easy to spread – the fact remains that hydrogenating the fat permanently alters the structure of the fat molecules. This once good-quality vegetable oil now becomes a trans-fatty acid.

In addition to the hydrogenation process, these oils are also bleached, coloured, perfumed and flavoured, just to make them resemble our beloved butter.

TFAs are not only found in margarine, but in thousands of commercial products worldwide. Many products available to us contain highly processed fats, for example, cakes, biscuits, muffins, donuts, chocolates, french fries, potato crisps and pastries.

These fats are now recognised as being carcinogenic and obviously very detrimental to our health. Animal fats (saturated) have long been blamed for the damage so often caused by partially-hydrogenated oils. These oils start out as wholesome, natural vegetable oils, only to be chemically altered by man.

The fats humans consumed for hundreds of years were, almost always, saturated fats. The extraction of oils from foods such as corn and many seeds was not easily done and the intact, whole foods (root, leaf, nut, grain or seed) were consumed complete with antioxidants and natural fibre. The fats contained within these food sources did not have to be artificially processed or hydrogenated to protect their integrity because they were consumed in their whole state, preventing rancidity. Accusations against chemically stable saturated fats don't really make sense when you realise that our own cells are busy making saturated fatty acids all the time from excess carbohydrates and protein.

Unless oils are bottled in dark tinted glass and state the words 'unrefined' as well as 'cold-pressed' on the container, you can almost guarantee they have been exposed to high temperatures in processing. The term 'cold-pressed' refers to a method of extracting oil from its source (e.g. olive), without the use of heat or chemicals. Unfortunately, even this term can be a misrepresentation. Heat may be produced through friction of mechanical grinding in the process of extraction, therefore the term 'unrefined' is perhaps more reliable. It is self-explanatory: it means the oil has not been through any process of refining or hydrogenation, therefore retaining a high level of nutritional value. If oil is not cold-pressed, it has been subjected to high temperatures to extract it, therefore destroying any vitamins and nutrients the oil contained originally. The value of these products to a food manufacturing or processing company is the fact that they have a longer shelf-life, less waste, and, of course, more revenue!

We have been encouraged to consume these products for many years now, only to find they can increase the risk of heart disease, cancer and many other related health problems. It is unfortunate that food manufacturers, in favour of profit, often overlook quality! I am certain that we would understand any additional cost involved in purchasing the healthier alternative if we were made aware of the consequences. It would be a lot less expensive than the medical bills accumulated due to ill health.

The best oils to purchase are those with labels stating 'mechanically-pressed and unrefined'. If a manufacturer has gone to the trouble of producing a high quality oil with all the relevant processing requirements to retain the nutrients, it will certainly be stated quite clearly on the container. Light destroys oil 1000 times faster than oxygen, therefore correct packaging is crucial. The bottom line is to choose the least processed and the least likely to go rancid when it comes to fats and oils. When purchasing bottled oils, always ensure that:

- the containers are either opaque in colour or darkened glass
- oils are kept refrigerated prior to and after purchase
- oils are frozen to retain freshness until ready to open
- oils are used within 3–6 weeks of opening.

In 1990, the fast food chain of McDonalds was pressured to switch their cooking oils from beef tallow to partially-hydrogenated vegetable oil to promote a healthier diet. The percentage of saturated fat in their fries dropped from 49% to 24% due to this change, however, the percentage of TFAs rose from 5% to 42–48% and the total amount of fat in the fries rose from 17.6% to 27.9%! Recently McDonalds has again switched to an oil that has cut TFAs in half, yet the beef tallow was still the better option … that is if french fries are to be consumed at all. The average American diet comprises 10–20% of calories from TFAs with some individuals consuming as much as 60 grams per day! Partially hydrogenated fats commonly contain 30–53% TFAs.

Trans-fatty acid content of some popular foods:

French fried potatoes	40% TFAs
Cookies & crackers	30–50% TFAs
Donuts	35–40% TFAs

'Age spots'

Otherwise referred to as 'fleurs de cemetiere', translated, 'cemetery flowers'. They appear on the skin surface as brown pigmentation patches, often seen on the back of elderly people's hands. These are known commonly as 'age spots', therefore accepted as a 'normal' part of the ageing process. They actually form due to fatty-acid degeneration within the body, usually through lack of the anti-oxidants, vitamin E and selenium.

How much fat should I eat?

Dietary fat is not easy to over-consume when it is not accompanied by refined carbohydrates. Most high-fat foods are heavily laden with refined carbohydrates, such as deep fried chips, battered and fried fish, chocolates, pastries, pizza, ice-cream, cakes, biscuits, cheesecake.

Not many people are going to consume too much fat by taking a swig from the olive oil bottle or munching on a slab of butter!

You will discover that your fat consumption will be self-regulating once you are consuming real food!

From our daily intake, the small intestine is capable of digesting around 10 grams of fat per hour. Consuming 1–3 tablespoons (12–

15% of our total calories) in the form of EFAs can help to speed up the body's metabolism significantly.